DATE DUE

The cytokines are a heterogeneous family of proteins which act via cell surface receptors to regulate and modify cell growth and maturation. They are thus implicated in a wide variety of physiological and pathological mechanisms. Understanding their mode of action is an important step towards developing their potential as therapeutic agents. Already many are successfully used in the treatment of a range of clinical disorders, including cancers, viral diseases and disorders of the immune system.

This book focuses on those cytokines which have the greatest therapeutic potential and whose clinical applications have been tried and tested. Each chapter is concerned with a specific cytokine and begins with a brief account of the relevant physiology and pharmacology. The clinical applications are then covered in detail, with reference to clinical studies, outlining the uses and potential benefits of the cytokines and including data on toxicity and the effectiveness of treatment. Each chapter is written by a leading authority whose clinical experience and expertise provides a valuable insight into the use of cytokines as a therapeutic tool.

Cytokine Therapy is a clear and concise introduction to the world of cytokines and their application to the treatment of disease. Written by clinicians, for clinicians, it provides the basis for a practical understanding of the uses of this important group of molecules. It will be of interest to all clinicians and of particular value to trainees and researchers in oncology, haematology and immunology.

Cytokine Therapy

CYTOKINE THERAPY

Edited by

David W. Galvani
and John C. Cawley

University Department of Haematology,
University of Liverpool, UK

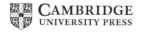

CAMBRIDGE
UNIVERSITY PRESS

Published by the Press Syndicate of the University of Cambridge
The Pitt Building, Trumpington Street, Cambridge CB2 1RP
40 West 20th Street, New York, NY 10011-4211, USA
10 Stamford Road, Oakleigh, Victoria 3166, Australia

First published 1992

Printed in Great Britain at the University Press, Cambridge

A catlogue record for this book is available from the British Library

Library of Congress Cataloging-in-Publication Data
Cytokine therapy / edited by David W. Galvani and John C. Cawley.
p. cm.
ISBN 0-521-41232-3 (hc). – ISBN 0-521-42337-6 (pb)
1. Cytokines – Therapeutic use. I. Galvani, David W. II. Cawley. J. C.
[DNLM: 1. Cytokines – therapeutic use. QW 568 C9945]
RM282.C95C97 1992
615'.7 – dc20
DNLM/DLC 92-16057 CIP

ISBN 0 521 41232 3 hardback
ISBN 0 521 42337 6 paperback

GE

CONTENTS

PREFACE

Cytokines are peptides that influence the growth and response of individual cells. Unlike hormones, they generally act in a localized manner on their target cells within a complex network, and they cannot be strictly utilized as 'hormone replacement'.

The field of cytokine research has grown exponentially over the past few years, resulting in an extensive scientific literature for each of the agents dealt with in the following chapters. This profusion of information is daunting for doctors and medical students, most of whom are already suffering from information overload. This book is a response to the requests of clinical colleagues who want an approachable and easily digestible account of those cytokines that are presently in clinical use. To this end, we have brought together a group of clinicians with extensive experience in the clinical use of each agent. The brief of each contributor was to provide a chapter containing two parts. The first part deals with the molecular and biological properties of each agent in a clear and concise manner. The second part summarizes the important clinical trial experience on a world-wide basis.

At the present time other agents such as interleukin-4 and interleukin-6 are undergoing clinical evaluation in humans, but there are insufficient data to place them with the others in this book. Yet other factors, e.g. transforming growth factor-ß, have major biological importance but are not presently available for assessment in man. This book has focused, therefore, on those cytokines that have been employed in extensive clincial studies and the reader is referred to the scientific literature and manuals on cytokine research for other agents.

We wish to acknowledge the efforts of each of the contributors in providing up to date material, and their patience during the editorial process.

D.W.G.
J.C.C.

LIST OF CONTRIBUTORS

Professor B B Aggarwal, Cytokine Research Laboratory, Department of Clinical Immunology and Biological Therapy, The University of Texas M D Anderson Cancer Center, 1515 Holcombe Boulevard, Houston, Texas 77030, USA

Professor G C Bagby, Jr, Division of Haematology & Medical Oncology, Oregon Health Sciences University and VA Medical Center, 3181 S W Sam Jackson Park Road, Portland, Oregon 97201-3098, USA

Professor M K Brenner, Department of Hematology-Oncology, St Judes Children's Research Hospital and University of Tennessee College of Medicine, 332 North Lauderdale, PO Box 318, Memphis, Tennessee 38101-0318, USA

Professor K Cantell, National Public Health Institute, Mannerheimintie 166, SF-00300 Helsinki, Finland

Professor J C Cawley, University Department of Haematology, 3rd Floor Duncan Building, Royal Liverpool University Hospital, PO Box 147, Liverpool L69 3BX, UK

Dr D W Galvani, University Department of Haematology, 3rd Floor Duncan Building, Royal Liverpool University Hospital, PO Box 147, Liverpool L69 3BX, UK

Dr A Ganser, Department of Haematology, Klinikum der Johann Wolfgang Goethe-Universitat, Theodor-Stern-Kai-7, 6000 Frankfurt a. M. 70, Germany

Professor D Hoelzer, Department of Haematology, Klinikum der Johann Wolfgang Goethe-Universitat, Theodor-Stern-Kai-7, 6000 Frankfurt a. M. 70, Germany

Dr K Huang, Department of Clinical Immunology & Biological Therapy, The University of Texas M D Anderson Cancer Center, 1515 Holcombe Boulevard, Houston, Texas 77030, USA

LIST OF CONTRIBUTORS

Dr A Khwaja, Department of Haematology, University College and Middlesex School of Medicine, 98 Chenies Mews, London WC1E 6HX, UK

Dr R Kurzrock, Department of Clinical Immunology and Biological Therapy, Box 41, M D Anderson Cancer Center, 1515 Holcombe Boulevard, Houston, Texas 77030, USA

Professor D C Linch, Department of Haematology, University College and Middlesex School of Medicine, 98 Chenies Mews, London WC1E 6HX, UK

Dr O G Ottmann, Department of Haematology, Klinikum der Johann Wolfgang Goethe-Universitat, Theodor-Stern-Kai-7, 6000 Frankfurt a. M. 70, Germany

Dr A A Rege, Texas Biotechnology Corp, 7000 Fannin St, Suite # 1810, Houston, Texas 77030, USA

Professor P M Sondel, Departments of Pediatrics and Human Oncology, University of Wisconsin Clinical Cancer Centre, 600 Highland Avenue, Madison, WI 53792, USA

Professor F Takaku, National Medical Centre Hospital, 1-21-1,Toyamacho, Shinjuku-ku, Tokyo 162, Japan

Dr C G Winearls, Renal Unit, Churchill Hospital and University of Oxford, Oxford OX3 7LJ, UK

1

INTRODUCTION: FROM INTERFERON RESEARCH TO CYTOKINE THERAPY

K. CANTELL

Interferons are forerunners in the cytokine field. They were the first cytokines to be discovered, they were the first cytokines to undergo clinical trials and they were the first cytokines to become registered drugs. This introductory chapter is a personal account by an old interferonologist, pondering whether something about the clinical application of cytokines at large can be learned from interferon research. It is dangerous to make generalizations, as some cytokines are pleiotropic whereas others are highly specific. However, some general principles derived from interferon research may also be applicable to other pleiotropic cytokines. The clinical application of specific cytokines, such as erythropoietin, is a different story.

Cytokines and biological response modifiers

What is a cytokine? It is not easy to define this rather heterogeneous group of protein cell regulators. All the substances described in this book are cytokines, but not all cytokines known at present are covered here. Are all protein growth factors cytokines? If not, which ones should be excluded from the cytokine club? All cytokines are 'biological response modifiers', but it is even more difficult to define a biological response modifier than to define a cytokine. Since, in my opinion, most drugs and other medical treatments could be said to affect biological responses, I will try to avoid this long, somewhat vague, term.

Towards increasing complexity

When interferon was first discovered (Isaacs and Lindenmann, 1957), it was thought to be a single, highly specific antiviral agent. Later work revealed

1

that there is not just a single interferon, but a whole superfamily of different interferons.

All interferons inhibit the multiplication of a wide range of different viruses. During the early years of interferon research, it was thought that interferons block a step common to the replication pathway of most viruses. Later work has revealed that the situation is far more complex. The multiplication of different viruses is inhibited at different stages of their replication cycle by one or more of the dozens of different proteins induced by interferon (Staeheli, 1990). The function of most of these proteins is completely unknown. Despite the early hopes, no unifying scheme has emerged; instead the picture has become ever more complex. I am afraid the same trend will hold for many other pleiotropic cytokines.

The pleiotropic nature of interferons was disclosed little by little, but even today, not much is known about their physiological roles. Are they primarily regulators of cell growth, cell division and differentiation? Are they primarily antiviral defence proteins? Why are there 15 different alpha interferons? Do they have specific functions? What are the main functions of beta and gamma interferons? Comprehension of the physiological roles of these proteins might aid in their clinical exploitation, but it is a very complicated task to unravel the roles of pleiotropic substances, entangled as they are in a complex network of positive and negative interactions between numerous cytokines. In their excellent book on cytokines, E. and J. de Maeyer (1988) quote the following insight of Rene Dubos: 'In the most common and probably the most important phenomena of life, the constituent parts are so interdependent that they lose their character, their meaning, and indeed their very existence when dissected from the functional whole'.

E. coli or human cell?

The clinical application of interferon was considered soon after its discovery. A broad spectrum of important diseases seemed to lend themselves as potential targets for interferon therapy. However, initial studies on the clinical front were painfully slow because interferon preparations suitable for clinical use were not available. The first systematic, small-scale clinical studies with interferon were begun some 15 years after its discovery. During the following decade, limited clinical trials were carried out with partially purified preparations of natural human leucocyte alpha interferons (Cantell, 1986). These studies indicated that, while interferon therapy can be effective against certain viral infections and tumours, it also has adverse effects. These findings aroused interest in interferon on the part of both clinicians and the general public, and pointed out the problems caused by the chronic shortage of interferon.

The cloning of the interferon genes (Nagata *et al.*, 1980; Taniguchi *et al.*, 1980) changed this situation, opening the way to obtaining precise information about the interferon genes and proteins and making mass production of these proteins possible. A few years later, the first recombinant alpha interferons became available for clinical use. This put an end to the shortage of interferon in principle, but in practice, some production problems have persisted. One of them concerns the host cell in which the interferon genes are expressed. Interferons and many other cytokines are currently produced for clinical use in *E. coli*. For example, all the commercially available recombinant alpha-2 interferon preparations are derived from *E. coli*. Their sequences differ with respect to one or two amino acids, and they are devoid of the carbohydrate groups of the natural alpha-2 interferon (Adolf *et al.*, 1991). It is not known whether these subtle structural differences are reflected in the clinical performance of the molecules, but it is clear that the recombinant alpha-2 interferons evoke antibodies in patients more often than does natural human leucocyte alpha interferon. Low levels of binding antibodies are not necessarily clinically harmful, but some patients develop high levels of neutralizing antibodies, which can abrogate the clinical efficacy of the recombinant products. This can result in a relapse, but in such patients remission can again be achieved with natural leucocyte alpha interferon (von Wussow *et al.*, 1989). This indicates that prokaryotic cells are not always ideal hosts for the production of cytokines for clinical purposes. For optimum clinical results, certain cytokines may have to be produced in eukaryotic cells, preferably in human cells.

The advent of recombinant DNA technology was of crucial importance for the mass production of cytokines for clinical purposes. However, one example from the field of interferon studies shows that, even today, there are alternative production systems. Those working with the production of human interferon in leucocyte suspensions in the 1960s realized, of course, that this method would never be suitable for true mass production. It was logical to look into immortal lymphoblastoid cell lines; some of these lines proved to be reasonably good producers of alpha interferons (Strander *et al.*, 1975). In the mid 1970s, Wellcome Biotechnology began studies with a lymphoblastoid cell line derived from a Ugandan child with Burkitt's lymphoma. An efficient production and purification procedure for lymphoblastoid alpha interferon was developed, clinical trials were started and the product was registered for clinical use at about the same time as the first recombinant alpha interferons. Thus human cell cultures can today be commercially competitive sources of cytokines for clinical use.

From laboratory to clinic

Herpetic keratitis is a superficial infection of the cornea caused by the herpes simplex virus. Studies on the topical interferon treatment of this important eye disease began in the early 1970s, when suitable interferon preparations became available. It took about ten years to learn how interferon should be used to obtain optimum results. Many disappointments were encountered along the way. For example, local application of interferon alone failed to prevent the recurrence of the disease or to improve its healing. However, when topical interferon was combined with a synthetic antiviral, such as trifluorothymidine or acyclovir, or with mechanical debridement, healing of the corneal ulcers was accelerated significantly (Sundmacher, 1982). Although these early studies have not received much publicity, I believe two lessons can be learned from them. First, it takes an amazing amount of time to find the optimal method for the clinical application of cytokines. In the seemingly simple case of herpetic keratitis, a decade was needed to establish an effective treatment schedule for topical interferon. If only interferon monotherapy had been tested, the erroneous conclusion would have been drawn that interferon is of no value in the treatment of this disease. Secondly, a cytokine which is ineffective on its own may still be highly effective in combination therapy. It may well be that cytokines, in general, work best in the presence of therapeutic partners.

With modern methods, cytokines can be quickly characterized and prepared for clinical studies. The pace of laboratory studies has accelerated greatly, but many scientists, not to speak of laymen, do not seem to understand fully that time spans in the clinic are very different. Sometimes much can be accomplished in the laboratory in weeks or months, whereas the clinical trials of cytokines inevitably take years.

Expectations and disappointments

Numerous articles have been written over the past years stating that interferon has been a clinical disappointment. This implies that the authors must have had great expectations for the clinical future of interferon. On the basis of laboratory and animal experiments, such expectations were hardly justified. I believe that, for those who have worked for a long time with interferon, its clinical performance has been a rather positive surprise. Alpha interferon, as the sole treatment, can keep hairy-cell leukaemia under control. Patients with certain solid tumours or chronic viral infections benefit from interferon monotherapy. Yet this is surely not the best way of exploiting interferons: their full clinical potentials will be realized in combination therapy.

Interferon received a great deal of publicity 10–15 years ago. The very limited availability and the high price of interferon increased its attraction. Unrealistic clinical hopes were raised. The publicity both helped and harmed research on interferon and cytokines. On the positive side, it increased pharmaceutical industry investments in interferon with the result that now, after several difficult years, interferon is becoming a billion-dollar drug. Although scientists tend to underrate financial aspects, in our market economy world, they have a strong impact on the future of any cytokine drug. Interferons have paved the way for other cytokines. Today, expectations for cytokine therapy are much more realistic than they had been a decade ago.

Future of cytokine therapy

Many new cytokines will surely be discovered, and clinical applications are likely to be found for all cytokines. Structural modification of the natural cytokines will yield a vast number of new drugs for clinical tests. Natural antagonists and man-made antagonists to different cytokines will also undergo clinical studies. All these biologicals must be tested in various combinations. Altogether, an almost endless variety of cocktails can be mixed from these ingredients.

Cytokines have come to the clinic to stay. Nothing will stop progress in this field, but no dramatic breakthroughs are foreseeable. Clinical results obtained with these physiological regulators are likely to improve in small steps. Infections and malignancies are the present main targets of cytokine therapy, but the spectrum of diseases treatable with cytokines is likely to expand.

Cytokine therapy has only just begun. Studies in this exciting field will continue for centuries.

REFERENCES

Adolf GR, Kalsner I, Ahorn H, Maurer-Fogy I and Cantell K (1991). Natural human interferon alpha-2 is O-glycosylated. *Biochemical J*. **276**, 511-18.

Cantell K (1986). Clinical performance of natural human leukocyte interferon. *Immunobiology*. **172**, 231-42.

de Maeyer E and de Maeyer J (1988). *Interferons and other regulatory cytokines*, 3-4. New York: John Wiley and Sons.

Isaacs A and Lindenmann J (1957). Virus interference. I. The interferon. *Proc Roy Soc*. **B147**, 258-67.

Nagata S, Taira H, Hall A *et al.* (1980). Synthesis in E. coli of a polypeptide with human leukocyte interferon activity. *Nature.* **284**, 316-20.

Staeheli P (1990). Interferon-induced proteins and the antiviral state. *Adv Vir Res.* **38**, 147-200.

Strander H, Mogensen KE and Cantell K. (1975). Production of human lymphoblastoid interferon. *J Clin Microbiol.* **1**, 116-17.

Sundmacher R (1982). Interferon in ocular diseases. In: *Interferon 4*, ed. Gresser I, 177-200. London: Academic Press.

Taniguchi T, Fujii-Kuriyama Y and Muramatsu M (1980). Molecular cloning of human interferon cDNA. *Proc Natl Acad Sci (USA).* **77**, 4003-6.

von Wussow P, Jakschies D, Freund M *et al.* (1989). Treatment of anti rIFN-alpha 2 antibody positive CML patients with natural interferon-alpha. *J Interferon Res.* **9**, S113.

2

ERYTHROPOIETIN

C. G. WINEARLS

INTRODUCTION

Of the haemopoietic growth factors available for clinical use, erythropoietin is the most widely used. The story of its discovery, purification and therapeutic application is a saga of starts, stops and serendipity (Erslev, 1991a). Perhaps most remarkable is the very short time it took after the cloning and expression of the human gene for the administration of the recombinant hormone to become part of routine clinical practice. The two papers describing cloning appeared in 1985 and it was later that year that Dr Joseph Eschbach treated the first patients in Seattle. The first clinical trials were completed within a year, the drug received its first licence in June 1988, and was available worldwide by 1989. This rapid development is explained in part by the fact that much was already known about the properties of the native hormone and the deficiency state in patients with chronic renal failure. Treatment of the anaemia of chronic renal failure is now routine so the focus of clinical research has changed from physiological replacement treatment to pharmacological use in an attempt to reverse other anaemias (Erslev, 1991b).

PHYSIOLOGY OF ERYTHROPOIETIN PRODUCTION

Erythropoietin is a true hormone (i.e. it is produced at one site but acts at another), the function of which is to maintain the red cell mass at a level to ensure optimal oxygen delivery to the tissues. Tissue oxygenation is determined by many other factors, including blood flow, the oxygen affinity and saturation of haemoglobin, the latter depending on the alveolar oxygen tension. The homeostatic function of erythropoietin is fulfilled by its action on

7

the erythroid marrow stimulating it to produce new red cells to replace the 1% of cells that reach the end of their 120-day lifespan each day. Under normal circumstances secretion of the hormone is at a low level maintaining plasma concentrations of 10–20 mIU/ml. There is a remarkable reserve capacity in response to hypoxia: plasma levels can rise 1000-fold and increase the rate of red cell production 5-fold.

Erythropoietin is produced mainly by the kidneys but small quantities are produced by the liver. The kidney seems an odd place for the production of a hormone that regulates the erythroid marrow. However, the kidney also acts as the oxygen sensor and in this role it is almost ideal for it is an organ with a high oxygen consumption, not subject to major fluctuations in demand or delivery but containing steep gradients which allow accurate 'reading' of the overall level of oxygen delivery. The nature of the oxygen sensor remains a mystery but there is an intriguing hypothesis that it is a haem protein which triggers erythropoietin production by adopting a de-oxy configuration when the cell is exposed to hypoxia (Goldberg et al., 1988). The search is now on to identify the elements of the erythropoietin gene complex that dictate expression in kidney and liver, and the sites at which factors produced in response to hypoxia bind to trigger transcription (Caro et al., 1991; Imagawa et al., 1991).

Which cells in the kidney produce erythropoietin? The clearest evidence comes from the experiments of Stephen Koury and his co-workers (Koury et al., 1988, 1989). They made mice anaemic (haematocrits ~15%) by bleeding and then sought the site of erythropoietin production by localizing its mRNA by in situ hybridization of a ^{35}S-labelled RNA probe complementary to the mRNA coding for erythropoietin. Cells containing erythropoietin mRNA were found primarily in the cortex of the kidney but not in the glomeruli. By careful destaining of the haematoxylin and eosin sections containing the emulsion and the silver grains, restaining with periodic acid Schiff, and photomicrographing the same area they were able to show that the positive cells always lay outside the tubular basement membrane. This suggested that the erythropoietin-producing cells were either a subset of interstitial cells or capillary endothelial cells.

THE ACTION OF ERYTHROPOIETIN

The maintenance of a constant red cell mass depends on the continual replacement of effete red cells or a compensatory increase in production if the loss of cells is accelerated. The original source is a stem cell that provides precursors for the whole of haemopoiesis including the erythroid progenitors.

It is the maturation and terminal differentiation and maintenance of viability of these that depends on erythropoietin (Koury and Bondurant, 1990; Adamson, 1991).

Erythropoietin acts on its target cells via a specific receptor expressed on the cell surface at a relatively low concentration (300–1000 receptors per cell). It belongs to a cytokine receptor super family which includes the receptors for interleukin-3 (IL-3), interleukin-4 (IL-4), interleukin-6 (IL-6), granulocyte-macrophage colony-stimulating factor (GM-CSF), prolactin and growth hormone. The greatest homology between these receptors is in their intracytoplasmic domains, suggesting that they have a common signal transduction mechanism. This mechanism has not been identified but the action of these growth factors is both to trigger proliferation and maintain viability of their target cells (D'Andrea and Zon, 1990).

The earliest identifiable component of the erythroid lineage that requires erythropoietin is the primitive burst-forming-unit-erythroid (BFU-E). To develop in marrow culture it also requires so-called burst-promoting-activity (BPA) which includes GM-CSF, IL-3, IL-4 and IL-6. Next is the mature BFU-E, which overlaps with the colony-forming-unit-erythroid (CFU-E) the most erythropoietin-sensitive erythroid progenitor.

RECOMBINANT HUMAN ERYTHROPOIETIN

This subject has recently been reviewed by Egrie and Browne (1991) and Hirth et al. (1988).

The native hormone was first purified in 1977 (Miyake et al., 1977), a step that provided material for partial peptide sequencing and the production of oligonucleotide probes with which to isolate the gene from both a cDNA and lambda bacteriophage human genomic DNA library (Jacobs et al., 1985; Lin et al., 1985). The gene has been expressed in Chinese hamster ovary cells which allow bulk culture and purification of the recombinant hormone in now limitless quantities.

The human gene (consisting of five exons and four introns) encodes a 193-amino-acid molecule from which a 27-amino-acid leader peptide and a C-terminal arginine are removed to yield a 165-amino-acid polypeptide (molecular weight 18.2 kDa) which undergoes glycosylation at four sites so that the final product has a molecular weight of 30.4 kDa. The glycosylation is required for secretion and confers stability on the molecule in vivo, preventing both aggregation and its rapid clearance by the liver via hepatic galactose receptors. The recombinant protein must therefore be produced in a mammalian cell line rather than in a bacterium or yeast, which cannot perform this post-translational modification. Although there may be subtle differences in the glycosylation between the native and recombinant forms of erythropoietin they are immunologically indistinguishable. There has so far been no report in humans of development of antibodies to the recombinant hormone. Two recombinant erythropoietins are now available for clinical use and these have been designated epoetin-alfa (Eprex®) and epoetin-beta (Recormon®) in the UK.

Clinical trials of epoetin proceeded without precise information on the pharmacokinetics after intravenous injection being available and one included studies of plasma half-life in the protocol (Cotes et al., 1989). Because no predictions of the relation between pharmacokinetics and pharmacodynamics could be made it was decided to administer epoetin by bolus i.v. injection to ensure delivery of the full dose and a high plasma concentration albeit transiently.

There are now a number of published reports of investigation of plasma clearance of intravenously administered epoetin in man (Spivak and Cotes, 1991). Estimates of the mean duration of the elimination phase vary from 4 to 12 h, with only a slight difference between subjects with normal renal function and those with renal failure. Subcutaneous administration will be the route of choice for most patients and is probably more effective unit for unit than the intravenous route (Bommer et al.,1988a; Muirhead and Wong, 1990). The pharmacokinetics are quite different. The peak concentration reached in the plasma is lower, ~4%, delayed, ~18 h, and prolonged. The bioavailability is ~20% of the intravenous dose (Macdougall et al., 1989; Hughes et al., 1989; Salmonson, 1990).

Intraperitoneal administration would only be suitable for patients maintained by Continuous Ambulatory Peritoneal Dialysis (CAPD) but there are no advantages in using this route in terms of efficacy or convenience (Macdougall et al., 1989; Lui et al., 1990; Frenken et al., 1990).

THE CLINICAL USE OF EPOETIN

Anaemia of chronic renal failure

Erythropoietin deficiency is a sufficient if not exclusive explanation for the anaemia of patients with chronic renal failure. Serum concentrations are within or slightly above the normal range but well below those found in patients with a comparable degree of anaemia but normal renal function (Caro et al., 1979).

It seems that the damaged kidney has a lower set point for erythropoietin production for although erythropoietin levels are inappropriately low for the degree of anaemia they do rise briskly in response to hypoxic stress (Walle *et al.*, 1987; Chandra *et al.*, 1988).

The fact that the rate of erythropoiesis is subnormal in renal failure patients despite the presence of normal concentrations of erythropoietin implies that the marrow is relatively hyporesponsive to erythropoietin. Evidence for depressed erythropoiesis includes: a reduced reticulocyte index, a decreased erythroid:granulocyte ratio in the bone marrow and a subnormal erythron transferrin uptake (ETU). The lower than normal rate of red cell production combined with an accelerated rate of red cell destruction is sufficient to set the steady state red cell mass at a lower level than normal. If the kidneys increase their erythropoietin production to a slightly higher level (e.g. if they develop acquired cystic disease), both these factors are overridden and the haemoglobin rises (Edmunds *et al.*, 1991).

There are unfortunately other factors, some of them in part avoidable, which operate in dialysis patients and conspire to aggravate the anaemia of chronic renal failure. These include: chronic intermittent blood loss, intercurrent infections, aluminium overload and iron deficiency.

Epoetin was first tested in haemodialysis patients with severe anaemia for which no cause other than renal failure could be found (Winearls *et al.*, 1986; Eschbach *et al.*, 1987; Cotes *et al.*, 1989). It was administered intravenously not only for convenience but also to ensure that high plasma concentrations similar to those seen in anaemic patients without renal failure were achieved.

The London Oxford Study (Winearls *et al.*, 1986; Reid *et al.*, 1988; Stevens *et al.*, 1989; Cotes *et al.*, 1989) included 15 haemodialysis patients with severe anaemia without confounding clinical problems. All responded, and the need for transfusions was abolished in the four who had previously been dependent on regular blood transfusion. The total red cell volume, which was below normal before treatment (mean = 8.9 ml/kg for the transfusion-dependent patients and 14.1 ml/kg in the seven non-transfused patients) increased following treatment to 24.2 ml/kg and 26 ml/kg respectively. Red cell survival in the seven non-transfused patients, which was only modestly shortened, was not altered by treatment and there was no overall correlation between red cell lifespan and maintenance dose requirements. The erythron transferrin uptake (ETU), an accurate measure of the erythroid marrow activity, derived from the plasma iron turnover, was subnormal in all but one case and following treatment an overall 2-fold increase was observed.

The response of bone marrow erythroid progenitors to rhEPO treatment was studied in nine of the subjects. Following treatment bone marrow BFU-E fell below pretreatment values but there was no significant change in the

CFU-E numbers. The fall in BFU-E can be explained by depletion of this compartment by erythropoietin-driven maturation to CFU-E without a commensurate replenishment from the pluripotential stem cell pool. The failure of the CFU-E numbers to change would then have to be explained by self-renewal and replenishment by BFU-E keeping the size of this compartment constant. The mitotic rate (percentage of cells in S-phase) was examined using the tritiated thymidine suicide technique and showed an increase for both CFU-E and BFU-E.

In the Seattle study (Eschbach et al., 1987) a range of doses between 1.5 and 1500 U/kg three times weekly were tested and this showed that the rate of rise in haemoglobin was dose-dependent and that the threshold dose for a response was 15 U/kg.

As soon as the efficacy of epoetin was established a number of large multicentre clinical trials were started.

1. The results of a European Multicentre Study of intravenous epoetin-alfa co-ordinated by Cilag Ltd were reported in November 1989 (Sundal and Kaeser, 1989) and updated in 1991 (Winearls et al., 1991). One-hundred-and-sixty-nine haemodialysis patients (mean pretreatment haemoglobin 7.0 g/dl) were entered into this study, of whom 163 were eligible for analysis. One-hundred-and-sixty-two responded (i.e. a rise in haemoglobin of > 2 g/dl). Of the 161 patients eligible for analysis for full response (reaching a target haemoglobin of 10–12 g/dl), 90% had done so by 16 weeks and all but two by 42 weeks. One-hundred-and-twenty-six patients were followed for at least one year and in these the maintenance dose required to keep within the target haemoglobin was shown to depend on the pretreatment level: Hb < 6 g/dl, 250–300 U/kg/week; Hb 6–8g/dl, 200 U/kg/week; Hb > 8 g/dl, 150–200 U/kg/week.

2. Later in the same year Eschbach and colleagues reported the results of the Amgen Phase III multicentre clinical trial of epoetin-alfa (Eschbach et al., 1989a). Three-hundred-and-thirty-three anaemic haemodialysis patients (mean haematocrit 0.223) received epoetin in doses of either 300 U/kg or 150 U/kg i.v. thrice weekly and then had the dose adjusted aiming for a target haematocrit of 0.35. Over 97% of the patients reached the target within 12 weeks. The median weekly maintenance dose was 225 U/kg/week.

3. The results of the European trials of epoetin-beta have been reported by a number of authors (Koch et al., 1988) and summarized by Bommer (Bommer et al., 1988b; Winearls et al., 1991). The patients were randomized to receive 40, 80 or 120 U/kg i.v. thrice weekly for 12 weeks after which the dose was adjusted to aim for a target haematocrit of 30–35%. Patients in all three groups responded but the rate of rise in haematocrit was significantly lower in the low dose group (40 U/kg). Investigators varied the dose frequency in the

maintenance phase and it emerged that the total dose was lower in those patients on thrice weekly injections (median dose 90 U/kg/week) compared to 160 U/kg in those on once or twice weekly dosing.

4. Several studies of the use of epoetin in CAPD patients have been completed and reported (Hughes *et al.*, 1990; Lui *et al.*, 1990; Macdougall *et al.*, 1990c; Piraino and Johnston, 1990; Stevens *et al.*, 1991). Macdougall *et al.* treated 15 severely anaemic patients with subcutaneous epoetin-beta, 10 of whom responded with an increase in haemoglobin to between 10 and 12 g/dl. In four of the five poor responders additional causes of anaemia were identified. Biochemical parameters and peritoneal function were unaffected by treatment. In the study reported by Stevens *et al.* 16 anaemic CAPD patients (Hb < 9 g/dl) were treated with thrice weekly subcutaneous epoetin-alfa, formulated at 10,000 IU/ml. The dose was adjusted to induce a stepwise increase in haemoglobin. Fourteen patients reached a target Hb of 11.0–11.5 g/dl and eight of these a second of 13.0–13.5 g/dl but one could not be maintained at this level. The median dose required to maintain the haemoglobin at 11.0–11.5 g/dl was 75 U/kg/week and at 13.0–13.5 g/dl was 150 U/kg/week. The conclusions from both studies were that twice or thrice weekly subcutaneous doses of epoetin are a well tolerated, convenient and effective treatment for anaemia in patients on CAPD and that the use of the intraperitoneal route is likely to be uneconomic and unnecessarily complicated.

5. Although the prevalence of severe anaemia is lower in patients with chronic renal failure not yet requiring dialysis (predialysis patients) it is nevertheless a cause of significant morbidity. When the trials were started in 1987 the particular question was whether raising the haematocrit would have an adverse effect on residual renal function. The double-blind placebo-controlled trial undertaken in the USA provides reassurance on this point (US Recombinant Human Erythropoietin Predialysis Study Group, 1991). No acceleration in the rate of decline in renal function has been observed. Moreover, subcutaneous administration of epoetin is as effective in inducing a response and maintaining a target haematocrit (Eschbach *et al.*, 1989b).

6. Rather fewer children than adults have been treated with epoetin. Their response and adverse experiences are similar but there was no evidence that treatment improved the growth of the treated children (Scigalla, 1991).

Although nephrologists are convinced of the benefits of epoetin treatment, a substantial body of objective evidence has accumulated. The most obvious benefit is the avoidance of blood transfusions. In the large Amgen trial described previously (Eschbach *et al.*, 1989a) the need for transfusions was abolished by 2 months. In this cohort of 333 patients there had been a requirement for 1030 units of blood in the 6 months prior to treatment (0.52

units per patient per month). Stopping regular transfusions will reduce the risk of transmission of hepatitis C and stop iron overload. In fact it is now possible to reverse established transfusion siderosis by venesecting patients treated with epoetin (Lazarus *et al.*, 1990). It is not yet clear what effect the change in transfusion practice will have on the results of renal transplantation. Stopping regular transfusions has been reported to reduce the breadth and titre of anti-HLA antibodies in sensitized patients in one study (Grimm *et al.*, 1990) but this was not confirmed by another group (Koskimies *et al.*, 1990).

The most comprehensive and rigorous evaluation of the effect of epoetin treatment on the quality of life of haemodialysis patients was undertaken by investigators in Canada (Canadian Erythropoietin Study Group, 1990). This was a double-blind study in which 40 patients were randomized to receive placebo, 40 to receive epoetin to achieve a haemoglobin of 9.5–11 g/dl and 38 a haemoglobin of 11.5–13 g/dl. Three different measures of 'quality of life' and assessments of exercise capacity were used. Compared with the placebo group the treated patients had significant improvements in their scores for fatigue and physical symptoms and an increase in the distance walked during a stress test. There was no improvement in the 6-min walk test, the psychosocial scores in the sickness impact profile or the time trade-off scores. Furthermore, there was no difference in exercise capacity between the two target haemoglobin groups.

Epoetin was initially licensed for intravenous administration and the recommended twice or thrice weekly bolus i.v. injections have the merit of simplicity and ensuring compliance in haemodialysis patients. However, subcutaneous (s.c.) injection would seem to provide a more physiological delivery of the hormone to the erythroid marrow. There is evidence (Bommer *et al.*, 1988a; Eschbach *et al.*, 1989b; Muirhead and Wong, 1990) that, despite the lower bioavailability of subcutaneous epoetin, it is, per unit dose, at least as, if not more, effective in stimulating erythropoiesis than i.v. epoetin. Preliminary data on the largest randomized comparison of i.v. and s.c. epoetin are available (Muirhead and Wong, 1990). One-hundred-and-twenty-eight dialysis patients were randomized to either 150 U/kg/week i.v. or s.c. with dose adjustments aiming for a target haemoglobin of 10.5–12.5 g/dl. The group receiving epoetin s.c. reached the target earlier than the i.v. group (12.9 $\pm$ 4.4 weeks versus 15.7 $\pm$ 3.8 weeks) and despite similar haemoglobin concentrations required lower maintenance doses (148 $\pm$ 122 U/kg/week versus 218 $\pm$ 104 U/kg/week).

There is evidence that daily low-dose s.c. epoetin administration may be the most economical treatment regimen (Granolleras *et al.*, 1989). If this proves to be the case patients will need formulations similar to insulin to simplify self-administration.

Now that epoetin is widely used nephrologists are not infrequently confronted by patients who fail to respond or who require particularly high doses. The most common explanation is iron deficiency (Eschbach et al., 1989a; Van Wyck et al., 1989). This is likely to develop if the ferritin concentration is < 100 mcg/l and will manifest as a waning response, with a falling transferrin saturation and ferritin concentration. Recently Macdougall et al. (1990b) have shown that the appearance of a population of hypochromic cells identified by an automated cell counter can provide an early clue. The recognition of aluminium overload is more subtle, requiring a desferrioxamine challenge test to estimate the aluminium burden and then treatment to remove this metal (Rosenlöf et al., 1990; Zachée et al., 1990). Dialysis patients are subject to a wide range of infections, some obvious and others occult and these are a frequent cause of a reduction in the haemoglobin concentration in patients established on treatment (Adamson and Eschbach, 1989; Muirhead and Hodsman, 1990; Stevens et al., 1991).

It was at first difficult to separate which of the adverse events experienced by patients receiving epoetin were coincidental, which were directly related to administration and which were a consequence of changes in haematocrit. A small number of patients (~ 4%) have reported flu-like symptoms after administration of the material (Winearls et al., 1986; Sundal and Kaeser, 1989; Eschbach et al., 1989a) but the Canadian placebo-controlled study found no difference in the numbers reporting this symptom (Canadian Erythropoietin Study Group, 1990). This may be accounted for by the fact that the initial reports were in patients receiving high doses as a rapid bolus which was not the case in the Canadian study. This side-effect was not reported by patients receiving epoetin subcutaneously (Stevens et al., 1991).

In about one-third of treated patients there is a clinically significant rise in blood pressure, which has been attributed to an increase in peripheral resistance following the relief of hypoxic dilatation and an increase in whole blood viscosity (Eschbach et al., 1989a; Eschbach, 1989; Sundal and Kaeser, 1989). In some of the early trials (Edmunds et al., 1989) there was a disturbing incidence of hypertensive encephalopathy and seizures. Reports of this are now much less frequent, perhaps because reversal of anaemia is being effected more slowly and clinicians are responding immediately to any changes in blood pressure.

There does seem to be a slightly higher incidence of vascular access failure after increasing the haemoglobin but this is often in access sites with pre-existing problems (Winearls et al., 1986; Sundal and Kaeser, 1989; Canadian Erythropoietin Study Group, 1990). Small increases in predialysis concentrations of creatinine, phosphate and potassium have been observed.

Table 2.1. *Recommendations for the use of recombinant human erythropoietin in patients with renal failure (prepared by the Executive Committee of the Renal Association, March 1990)*

Groups of patients to be treated
i   Patients requiring regular blood transfusion ii Patients with angina or heart failure aggravated by anaemia iii Patients with haemoglobin concentrations < 8 g/dl iv Patients whose livelihoods are threatened by anaemia v   Patients in whom transfusion is to be avoided to reduce sensitization to transplantation antigens

Apart from potassium (Eschbach *et al.*, 1987) these were not usually clinically significant and probably reflect changes in diet and dialysis efficiency (Casati *et al.*, 1987; Sundal and Kaeser, 1989; Eschbach *et al.*, 1989a).

An important and unresolved issue is that of the optimal target haemoglobin concentration for which to aim. For patients accustomed to a haemoglobin of < 8 g/dl a rise to 10 g/dl would be welcome but what should the target be for the younger and more athletic patients? Can such patients notice a difference between a haemoglobin of 10 and 13 g/dl? The Canadian study which compared the quality of life in two groups of patients at different target haemoglobins (9.5–11 g/dl and 11.5–13 g/dl) found no significant difference in the improvement in quality of life or exercise capacity between the two groups. There is a belief among many nephrologists that achieving a normal haemoglobin concentration will be associated with a higher risk of side-effects including hypertension and vascular access failure. This, plus the higher dose, and therefore cost of maintaining a normal haemoglobin concentration, has led to a target of 10–12 g/dl being generally accepted.

Treatment with epoetin is, in comparison with other drugs, expensive. In the UK an ampoule of 4000 units costs £36 ($61) excluding VAT. The cost of treating individual patients depends on their weight, the target haemoglobin and their responsiveness. At an average dose requirement of 150 U/kg/week the annual cost would be about £4000 ($6800) per annum but subcutaneous administration and a lower target haemoglobin may reduce this. Because of concerns of cost the Renal Association in UK prepared guidelines on the use of erythropoietin (Table 2.1) which were endorsed by the Department of

Health. In the USA an ad hoc committee of the National Kidney Foundation simply recommended that, 'patients with renal failure and haematocrits that remain lower than 30% without transfusions are eligible for epo therapy' (the Ad Hoc Committee of the National Kidney Foundation, 1989). More general guidelines on treatment have been set out by the Cardiff erythropoietin research group (Macdougall et al., 1990a).

Prematurity

Anaemia is common in premature neonates and many require blood transfusions. The normal physiological fall in haemoglobin concentration that occurs after delivery is exaggerated in premature infants and the demands placed on the erythroid marrow are substantial for their red cells have a shortened lifespan and they are in a phase of rapid growth. The problem is compounded by frequent blood sampling for laboratory tests. Five millilitres a day taken for this purpose would remove 75% of the red cell mass in 1 week. Although there is no deficiency in erythroid precursors or their sensitivity to erythropoietin (Shannon et al., 1987) the erythroid marrow does not keep up with the demands placed upon it. This failure is in part a consequence of inadequate erythropoietin secretion by the immature kidneys (Brown et al., 1984) suggesting a physiological basis for treating premature neonates with recombinant erythropoietin. In the studies of epoetin treatment of premature neonates that have been reported (Halperin et al., 1990; Obladen et al., 1991; Shannon et al., 1991) the effects have been either absent or minimal, but it may be that the doses used were inadequate.

Autologous transfusion

The use of autologous blood to cover surgery has three advantages: (1) it reduces the risk of transmission of infections such as hepatitis, (2) it reduces the demand placed on the blood bank and (3) it avoids the problems of finding blood for patients with red cell antibodies who are difficult to crossmatch. Goodnough et al. (1989) have shown that the administration of epoetin (600 U/kg twice weekly) during the period of blood collection allows more blood to be harvested and a higher haematocrit to be maintained. At this dose the treatment is costly (£2000; $3400) making the extra units of blood obtained unacceptably expensive. It may be possible to modify the protocol, e.g. by administering epoetin subcutaneously and starting treatment earlier. At present its use can only be justified in patients in whom heterologous blood transfusion is to be avoided or is impossible (Green and Handley, 1990; Rothstein *et al.*, 1990).

Rheumatoid arthritis

Anaemia is a common feature of chronic infection and inflammation. The pathophysiology is complex but a number of abnormalities have been identified. Red cell survival is shortened, the release of iron by the reticuloendothelial system is impaired and the marrow is suppressed (Erslev, 1985). Although the erythropoietin levels are raised, the concentrations may be lower than expected and certainly do not exert an adequate response from the marrow. Despite the controversy over whether erythropoietin concentrations are, or are not appropriate for the degree of anaemia (Baer *et al.*, 1987; Birgegård *et al.*, 1987; Hochberg *et al.*, 1988), rheumatoid arthritis was the obvious chronic inflammatory condition in which to test the effect of epoetin.

The results of a placebo-controlled multicentre study were published in 1990 (Pincus *et al.*, 1990). Seventeen patients with rheumatoid arthritis and haematocrits < 34% and without obvious additional causes of anaemia such as renal disease or bleeding, were randomized to receive placebo or epoetin (50, 100, 150 U/kg i.v. thrice weekly) for 8 weeks, after which the study was opened and all patients could receive active treatment and the dose adjusted. By the end of the eight-week treatment period only 4/13 of the epoetin-treated patients had responded (an increase in haematocrit of six points) but none of the placebo group had done so. In the open phase all eight patients receiving treatment responded so that overall there were 12/16 responders. Although the result of the placebo-controlled phase of the study appears rather disappointing, the outcome in the open phase shows that this anaemia is reversible by exogenous epoetin. There are as yet insufficient data to say whether the doses required are higher than those needed by patients with renal failure.

The careful evaluation of these patients revealed that many had previously unrecognized iron deficiency but all were treated with oral iron and none responded to this alone. Although no side-effects of treatment were observed no benefits, e.g. improved activity, were detected either. This and other studies (Takashina *et al.*, 1990) suggest that although epoetin treatment can override the inflammatory mediators of anaemia, treatment should be offered only to those patients in whom anaemia is actually causing symptoms; in whom other causative factors, especially iron deficiency have been excluded

(Vreugdenhil *et al.*, 1990) and in whom the underlying disease cannot be controlled with anti-inflammatory agents.

Cancer and haematological malignancy

This subject was recently reviewed by Bunn (1990).

The treatment of anaemia in patients with malignant disease with epoetin does not at first seem rational. There are multiple and synergistic factors contributing to its causation and, although erythropoietin levels are lower than would be predicted for the degree of anaemia (Miller *et al.*, 1990) this blunting is not that striking and certainly does not resemble that seen in patients with renal disease. The combination of marrow infiltration, blood loss, chemotherapy, whatever mechanisms operate in the anaemia of chronic disease and rarely autoimmune haemolysis represents a formidable bar to the physiological action of erythropoietin. This pessimistic background notwithstanding, the results from pilot studies are encouraging.

Oster and colleagues (1990) treated five anaemic patients with non-Hodgkin's lymphoma and extensive bone marrow infiltration and elevated concentrations of endogenous erythropoietin with an rhEPO produced from a murine fibrosarcoma cell line, at doses of 300–900 U/kg/week. Four patients responded and became independent of transfusions.

There is an encouraging report of the amelioration of anaemia in a patient with chronic lymphocytic leukaemia, 72% marrow infiltration and transfusion dependence, treated with 4000 units of epoetin-alfa three times weekly. The effect was particularly welcome because the patient had developed red cell antibodies, which made finding compatible blood difficult (Davis and Brown, 1991). There may, however, be a problem with treating patients with leukaemia and myelofibrosis. Two such cases developed fever and increasing splenomegaly, attributed to extramedullary erythropoiesis, after epoetin treatment (Iki *et al.*, 1991).

Despite the usually very high levels of plasma erythropoietin there are reports of improvements in anaemia in a few patients with myelodysplastic syndromes treated with epoetin (Stebler *et al.*, 1990; Bowen *et al.*, 1991).

The anaemia of patients with multiple myeloma is caused by a combination of bone marrow infiltration, chemotherapy, infection and renal failure. Nielsen *et al.* (1990) have measured serum erythropoietin levels in patients with myeloma and found that they were appropriate in anaemic non-uraemic subjects but not in those with renal failure. Taylor *et al.* have described the successful reversal of anaemia, with standard doses of epoetin, in patients with myeloma and end-stage renal failure maintained by dialysis. Presumably the predominant cause of the anaemia in these cases was erythropoietin deficiency from renal failure (Taylor et al., 1990) for no details of the degree of marrow infiltration at the time of epoetin treatment were given. What was more surprising was the report of Ludwig et al. (1990) who treated thirteen patients with multiple myeloma who had normal plasma creatinine concentrations. Eleven had a steady increase in haemoglobin and reversal of anaemia. The non- and late-responders had higher erythropoietin concentrations than the responders, suggesting that their anaemia was not related to a relative deficiency of erythropoietin. There is an anxiety about treating such patients with a growth factor because of the possibility that some myelomas may be erythropoietin-dependent. Okuno et al. (1990) have described the expression of the erythropoietin receptor on a human myeloma cell line (MM1-S1) but they do not state whether the cells growth was dependent on the hormone. In the study reported by Ludwig et al. there was no evidence of a change in the behaviour of the myeloma during epoetin treatment, but Rogers et al. (1990) have reported a patient with renal failure treated with epoetin in whom there was a temporary increase in urinary excretion of a lambda light chain during treatment.

Epoetin treatment has a theoretically sound justification in those patients developing anaemia after cisplatinum treatment, as this agent is nephrotoxic and the anaemia-induced erythropoietin response is partly suppressed (Matsumoto et al., 1990). Trials of its use in this setting are in progress (Henry et al., 1989).

Anaemia in patients with AIDS

Patients with AIDS are liable to develop anaemia because of the direct effects of the virus on the marrow, the direct and indirect consequences of opportunistic infections, vitamin B_{12} deficiency, blood loss and the myelotoxic effect of azidothymidine (AZT) (Richman et al., 1987). There is also a blunted erythropoietin response to anaemia in patients with HIV infection (Spivak et al., 1989) but treatment with AZT which exacerbates anaemia is associated with a significantly 'better' erythropoietin response. This complicated interpretation of the first trial of epoetin treatment of anaemic AIDS patients treated with AZT (Fischl et al., 1990a). The trial was randomized, double-blind and placebo-controlled, the active treatment being 100 units/kg of epoetin-alfa i.v. thrice weekly for 12 weeks. A reduction in the number of transfusions required was seen only in the group with baseline endogenous erythropoietin concentrations < 500 mIU/ml. Later studies using higher doses of epoetin given subcutaneously have apparently confirmed this

ERYTHROPOIETIN

finding (Henry and Abels, 1991). Since these reports have appeared, lower doses of AZT have been shown to be as effective in the treatment of AIDS and associated with a reduced tendency to cause anaemia and neutropenia (Fischl *et al.*, 1990b). It seems, therefore, that epoetin will only be used in that small subset of transfusion-dependent AIDS patients with endogenous erythropoietin concentrations < 500 mIU/ml.

Other conditions

Epoetin has been used to accelerate recovery from post-partum anaemia (Danko *et al.*, 1990) but the benefits were modest. Its role in this circumstance will probably be to treat those patients who refuse blood transfusions.

Regrettably, epoetin will be used to enhance athletic performance – an abuse that will be rather difficult to prove.

REFERENCES

Ad Hoc Committee of the National Kidney Foundation (1989). Statement on the clinical use of recombinant erythropoietin in anemia of end-stage renal disease. *Am J Kid Dis.* **14**, 163–9.

Adamson JW (1991). The erythroid response to erythropoietin. In *Erythropoietin, molecular, cellular and clinical biology,* ed. AJ Erslev, JW Adamson, JW Eschbach and CG Winearls, 99–114. Baltimore: The Johns Hopkins University Press.

Adamson JW and Eschbach JW (1989). Management of the anaemia of chronic renal failure with recombinant erythropoietin. *Quart J Med.* **73**, 1093–101.

Baer AN, Dessypris EN, Goldwasser E *et al.* (1987). Blunted erythropoietin response to anaemia in rheumatoid arthritis. *Br J Haematol.* **66**, 559–64.

Birgegård G, Hällgren R and Caro J (1987). Serum erythropoietin in rheumatoid arthritis and other inflammatory arthritides: relationship to anaemia and the effect of anti-inflammatory treatment. *Br J Haematol.* **65**, 479–83.

Bommer J, Ritz E, Weinreich T *et al.* (1988a). Subcutaneous erythropoietin (letter). *Lancet.* **2**, 406.

Bommer J, Kugel M, Schoeppe W *et al.* (1988b). Dose-related effects of recombinant human erythropoietin on erythropoiesis. Results of a multicenter trial in patients with end-stage renal disease. *Contributions to Nephrology.* **66**, 85–93.

Bowen DT, Culligan D and Jacobs A (1991). The treatment of anaemia in the myelodysplastic syndromes with recombinant human erythropoietin. *Br J Haematol.* **77**, 419–23.

Brown MS, Garcia JF, Phibbs RH *et al.* (1984). Decreased response of plasma immunoreactive erythropoietin to "available oxygen" in anemia of prematurity. *J Ped.* **105**, 793–8.

Bunn HF (1990). Recombinant erythropoietin therapy in cancer patients. *J Clin Oncol.* **8**, 949–51.

Canadian Erythropoietin Study Group (1990). Association between recombinant human erythropoietin and quality of life and exercise capacity of patients receiving haemodialysis. *Br Med J.* **300**, 573–8.

Caro J, Brown S, Miller O *et al.* (1979). Erythropoietin levels in uremic nephric and anephric patients. *J Lab Clin Med.* **93**, 449–58.

Caro J, Beck I, Ramirez S *et al.* (1991). Regulation of erythropoietin gene expression. *Sem Hematol.* **28 (suppl 3)**, 42–6.

Casati S, Passerini P, Campise MR *et al.* (1987). Benefits and risks of protracted treatment with human recombinant erythropoietin in patients having haemodialysis. *Br Med J.* **295**, 1017–20.

Chandra M, Clemons GK and McVicar MI (1988). Relation of serum erythropoietin levels to renal excretory function: evidence for lowered set point for erythropoietin production in chronic renal failure. *J Ped.* **113**, 1015–21.

Cotes PM, Pippard MJ, Reid CDL *et al.* (1989). Characterization of the anaemia of chronic renal failure and the mode of its correction by a preparation of erythropoietin (r-HuEPO). An investigation of the pharmacokinetics of intravenous r-HuEPO and its effect on erythrokinetics. *Quart J Med.* **70**, 113–37.

D'Andrea AD and Zon LI (1990). Erythropoietin receptor. Subunit structure and activation. *J Clin Invest.* **86**, 681–7.

Danko J, Huch R and Huch A (1990). Epoetin alfa for treatment of postpartum anaemia (letter). *Lancet.* **335**, 737–8.

Davis HP and Brown H (1991). Epoetin alfa for anaemia of chronic leukaemia (letter). *Lancet.* **337**, 47.

Edmunds ME, Walls J, Tucker B *et al.* (1989). Seizures in haemodialysis patients treated with recombinant human erythropoietin. *Nephrol Dial Transplant.* **4**, 1065–9.

Edmunds ME, Devoy M, Tomson CRV *et al.* (1991). Plasma erythropoietin levels and acquired cystic disease of the kidney in patients receiving regular dialysis treatment. *Brit J Haematol.* **78**, 275–7.

Egrie JC and Browne JK (1991). The molecular biology of erythropoietin. In *Erythropoietin, molecular, cellular and clinical biology,* ed. AJ Erslev, JW Adamson, JW Eschbach and CG Winearls, 21–40. Baltimore: The Johns Hopkins University Press.

Erslev AJ (1985). Anemia of chronic disorders. In *Hematology*, 3rd edn, ed. WJ Williams, E Beutler, AJ Erslev and MA Lichtman, 522–8. New York: McGraw-Hill.

Erslev AJ (1991a). Erythropoietin: from physiology to clinical trials via molecular biology. In *Erythropoietin, molecular, cellular, and clinical biology*, ed. AJ

ERYTHROPOIETIN

Erslev, JW Adamson, JW Eschbach and CG Winearls, 3–18. Baltimore: The Johns Hopkins University Press.

Erslev AJ (1991b). Drug therapy: erythropoietin. *N Engl J Med.* **324**, 1339–44.

Eschbach JW (1989). The anaemia of chronic renal failure: Pathophysiology and effects of recombinant erythropoietin. *Kidney International.* **35**, 134–48.

Eschbach JW, Egrie JC, Downing MR *et al.* (1987). Correction of the anemia of end-stage renal disease with recombinant human erythropoietin. Results of a combined phase I and II clinical trial. *N Engl J Med.* **316**, 73–8.

Eschbach JW, Abdulhadi MH, Browne JK *et al.* (1989a). Recombinant human erythropoietin in anemic patients with end-stage renal disease. *Ann Int Med.* **111**, 992–1000.

Eschbach JW, Kelly MR, Haley RN *et al.* (1989b). Treatment of the anemia of progressive renal failure with recombinant human erythropoietin. *N Engl J Med.* **321**, 158–63.

Fischl M, Galpin JE, Levine JD *et al.* (1990a). Recombinant human erythropoietin for patients with AIDS treated with zidovudine. *N Engl J Med.* **322**, 1488–93.

Fischl MA, Galpin JE, Levine JD *et al.* (1990b). A randomised controlled trial of a reduced daily dose of zidovudine in patients with the acquired immunodeficiency syndrome. *N Engl J Med.* **323**, 1009–14.

Frenken LAM, Struijk LJ, Coppens PJW *et al.* (1990). Comparative study of intraperitoneal and subcutaneous administration of recombinant-human erythropoietin in patients treated with continuous ambulatory peritoneal dialysis. *Eur J Clin Invest.* **20**, A56.

Goldberg MA Dunning SP and Bunn FH (1988). Regulation of the erythropoietin gene: evidence that the oxygen sensor is a heme protein. *Science.* **242**, 1412–5.

Goodnough LT, Rudnick S, Price TH *et al.* (1989). Increased preoperative collection of autologous blood with recombinant human erythropoietin therapy. *N Engl J Med.* **321**, 1163–8.

Granolleras C, Branger B, Beau MC *et al.* (1989). Experience with daily self-administered subcutaneous erythropoietin. *Contrib Nephrol.* **76**, 143–8.

Green D and Handley E (1990). Erythropoietin for anemia in Jehovah's witness. *Ann Int Med.* **113**, 720–1.

Grimm PC, Sinai-Trieman L, Sekiya NM *et al.* (1990). Effects of recombinant human erythropoietin on HLA sensitization and cell mediated immunity. *Kidney International.* **38**, 12–18.

Halperin DS, Wacker P, Lacourt G *et al.* (1990). Effects of recombinant human erythropoietin in infants with the anemia of prematurity: A pilot study. *J Ped.* **116**, 779–86.

Henry DH and Abels RI (1991). Recombinant human erythropoietin (Epoetin-alfa) in patients with AIDS and AZT-induced anemia. In *Erythropoietin, molecular, cellular and clinical biology,* ed. AJ Erslev, JW Adamson, JW Eschbach and CG Winearls, 419–33. Baltimore: The Johns Hopkins University Press.

Henry DH, Rudnick SA and Bryant E *et al*. (1989). Preliminary report of two double blind, placebo controlled studies using recombinant human erythropoietin (rHuEpo) in the anaemia associated with cancer. *Blood*. **74**, 6a.

Hirth P, Wieczorek L and Scigalla P (1988). Molecular biology of erythropoietin. *Contrib Nephrol*. **66**, 38–53.

Hochberg MC, Arnold CM, Hogans BB *et al*. (1988). Serum immunoreactive erythropoietin in rheumatoid arthritis: impaired response to anemia. *Arthritis Rheum*. **31**, 1318–21.

Hughes RT, Cotes PM, Oliver DO *et al*. (1989). Correction of the anaemia of chronic renal failure with erythropoietin (r-HuEPO): pharmacokinetic studies during haemodialysis and CAPD. *Contrib Nephrol*. **76**, 122–30.

Hughes RT, Cotes PM, Pippard MJ *et al*. (1990). Subcutaneous administration of recombinant human erythropoietin to subjects on continuous ambulatory peritoneal dialysis: An erythrokinetic assessment. *Br J Haematol*. **75**, 268–73.

Iki S, Yagisawa M, Ohbayashi Y *et al*. (1991). Adverse effect of erythropoietin in myeloproliferative disorders (letter). *Lancet*. **337**, 187–8.

Imagawa S, Goldberg MA. Doweiko J *et al*. (1991). Regulatory elements of the erythropoietin gene. *Blood*. **77**, 278–85.

Jacobs K, Shoemaker C, Rudersdorf R *et al*. (1985). Isolation and characterisation of genomic and cDNA clones of human erythropoietin. *Nature*. **313**, 806–10.

Koch KM, Kühn K, Nonnast-Daniel B and Scigalla P (1988). Treatment of renal anemia with recombinant human erythropoietin. *Contrib Nephrol*. **66**, 5–20.

Koskimies S, Lautenschlager I, Grönhagen-Riska C *et al*. (1990). Erythropoietin therapy and the antibody levels of highly sensitized patients awaiting kidney transplantation. *Transplantation*. **50**, 707–9.

Koury MJ and Bondurant MC (1990). Erythropoietin retards DNA breakdown and prevents programmed death in erythroid progenitor cells. *Science*. **248**, 378–81.

Koury ST, Bondurant MC and Koury MJ (1988). Localization of erythropoietin synthesizing cells in murine kidneys by in situ hybridization. *Blood*. **71**, 524–7.

Koury ST, Koury MJ, Bondurant MC *et al*. (1989). Quantitation of erythropoietin-producing cells in kidneys of mice by in situ hybridization: correlation with haematocrit, renal erythropoietin mRNA, and serum erythropoietin concentration. *Blood*. **74**, 645–51.

Lazarus JM, Hakim RM and Newell J (1990). Recombinant human erythropoietin and phlebotomy in the treatment of iron overload in chronic hemodialysis patients. *Am J Kid Dis*. **16**, 101–8.

Lin FK, Suggs S, Lin CH *et al*. (1985). Cloning and expression of the human erythropoietin gene. *Proc Natl Acad Sci U.S.A*. **82**, 7580–4.

Ludwig H, Fritz E, Kotzmann H *et al*. (1990). Erythropoietin treatment of anemia associated with multiple myeloma. *New Engl J Med*. **322**, 1693–9.

Lui SF, Chung WWM, Leung CB *et al*. (1990). Pharmacokinetics and pharmacodynamics of subcutaneous and intraperitoneal administration of recombinant human erythropoietin in patients on continuous ambulatory peritoneal dialysis. *Clin Nephrol.* **33**, 47–51.

Macdougall IC, Roberts DE, Neubert P *et al.* (1989). Pharmacokinetics of recombinant human erythropoietin in patients on continuous ambulatory peritoneal dialysis. *Lancet.* **1**, 425–7.

Macdougall IC, Hutton RD, Cavill I *et al.* (1990a). Treating renal anaemia with recombinant human erythropoietin: practical guidelines and a clinical algorithm. *Br Med J.* **300**, 655–9.

Macdougall IC, Cavill I, Hulme B *et al.* (1990b). Detection of functional iron deficiency during epo therapy: a new approach. *J Am Soc Nephrol.* **1**, 402. (Abstract)

Macdougall IC, Davies ME, Hutton RD *et al.* (1990c). The treatment of renal anaemia in CAPD patients with recombinant human erythropoietin. *Nephrol Dial Transplant.* **5**, 950–5.

Matsumoto T, Endoh K, Kamisango K *et al.* (1990). Effect of recombinant human erythropoietin on anticancer drug-induced anaemia. *Br J Haematol.* **75**, 463–8.

Miller CB, Jones RJ, Piantadosi S *et al.* (1990). Decreased erythropoietin response in patients with the anemia of cancer. *N Engl J Med.* **322**, 1689–92.

Miyake T, Kung CK and Goldwasser E (1977). Purification of human erythropoietin. *J Biol Chem.* **252**, 5558–64.

Muirhead N and Hodsman AB (1990). Occult infection and resistance of anaemia to rHuEPO therapy in renal failure. *Nephrol Dial Transplant.* **5**, 232–234.

Muirhead N and Wong C (1990). Erythropoietin for anemia in high risk hemodialysis patients: comparison of iv and sc administration. *J Am Soc Nephrol.* **1**, 404. (Abstract)

Nielsen OJ, Brandt M and Drivsholm A (1990). The secretory erythropoietin response in patients with multiple myeloma and Waldenstrom's macroglobulinaemia. *Scan J Clini Lab Invest.* **50**, 697–703.

Obladen M, Maier R, Segerer H *et al.* (1991). Efficacy and safety of recombinant human erythropoietin to prevent the anemias of prematurity. European, randomised, multicenter trial. *Contrib Nephrol.* **88**, 314–26.

Okuno Y, Takahashi, T Suzuki A *et al.* (1990). Expression of the erythropoietin receptor on a human myeloma cell line. *Bioch Biophys Res Comm.* **170**, 1128–34.

Oster W, Herrmann F, Gamm H *et al.* (1990). Erythropoietin for the treatment of anemia of malignancy associated with neoplastic bone marrow infiltration. *J Clin Oncol.* **8**, 956–62.

Pincus T, Olsen NJ, Russell IJ *et al.* (1990). Multicenter study of recombinant human erythropoietin in correction of anemia in rheumatoid arthritis. *Am J Med.* **89**, 161–8.

Piraino B and Johnston JR (1990). The use of subcutaneous erythropoietin in CAPD patients. *Clin Nephrol.* **33**, 200–2.

Reid CDL, Fidler J, Oliver DO *et al.* (1988). Erythroid progenitor cell kinetics in chronic haemodialysis patients responding to treatment with recombinant human erythropoietin. *Br J Haematol.* **70**, 375–80.

Richman DD. Fischl MA, Grieco MH *et al.* (1987). The toxicity of azidothymidine (AZT) in the treatment of patients with AIDS and AIDS-related complex: a double-blind, placebo-controlled trial. *N Engl J Med.* **317**, 192–17.

Rogers S, Russell NH and Morgan AG (1990). Effect of erythropoietin in patients with myeloma. *Br Med J.* **301**, 667–9.

Rosenlöf K, Fyhrquist F and Tenhunen R (1990). Erythropoietin, aluminium, and anaemia in patients on haemodialysis. *Lancet.* **335**, 247–9.

Rothstein P, Roye D, Verdisco L *et al.* (1990). Preoperative use of erythropoietin in an adolescent Jehovah's Witness. *Anesthesiol.* **73**, 568–70.

Salmonson T (1990). Pharmacokinetic and pharmacodynamic studies on recombinant human erythropoietin. *Scan J Urol Nephrol.* **Suppl 129**, 1–66.

Scigalla P (1991). Recombinant human erythropoietin (epoetin-beta) in children with renal anaemia: Western Europe. In *Erythropoietin, molecular, cellular and clinical biology,* ed. AJ Erslev, JW Adamson, JW Eschbach and CG Winearls, 355–73. Baltimore: The Johns Hopkins University Press.

Shannon KM, Naylor GS, Torkildson JC *et al.* (1987). Circulating erythroid progenitors in the anemia of prematurity. *N Engl J Med.* **317**, 728–33.

Shannon KM, Mentzer WC, Abels RI *et al.* (1991). Recombinant human erythropoietin in anemia of prematurity: results of a placebo-controlled pilot study. *J Ped.* **118**, 949–55.

Spivak JL, Barnes DC, Fuchs E *et al.* (1989). Serum immunoreactive erythropoietin in HIV-infected patients. *J Am Med Assoc.* **261**, 3104–7.

Spivak JL and Cotes PM (1991). The pharmacokinetics and metabolism of erythropoietin. In *Erythropoietin, molecular, cellular and clinical biology,* ed. AJ Erslev, JW Adamson, JW Eschbach and CG Winearls, 162–83. Baltimore: The Johns Hopkins University Press..

Stebler C, Tichelli A, Dazzi H *et al.* (1990). High-dose recombinant human erythropoietin for treatment of anemia in myelodysplastic syndromes and paroxysmal nocturnal hemoglobinuria: A pilot study. *Expt Hematol.* **18**, 1204–8.

Stevens JM, Forman EW, Oliver DO *et al.* (1989). 18–24 months follow-up of chronic haemodialysis patients receiving recombinant human erythropoietin. *Nephrol Dial Transplant.* **3**, 501. (Abstract)

Stevens JM, Auer J, Strong CA *et al.* (1991). Stepwise correction of anaemia by subcutaneous administration of human recombinant erythropoietin (epoetin-alfa) in patients with chronic renal failure maintained by continuous ambulatory peritoneal dialysis. *Nephrol Dial Transplant.* **6**, 487–94.

Sundal E and Kaeser U (1989). Correction of anaemia of chronic renal failure with recombinant human erythropoietin: safety and efficacy of one year's treatment in a European Multicentre Study of 150 haemodialysis-dependent patients. *Nephrol Dial Transplant.* **4**, 979–87.

Takashina N, Kondo H and Kashiwazaki S (1990). Suppressed serum erythropoietin respomse to anemia and the efficacy of recombinant erythropoietin in the anemia of rheumatoid arthritis. *J Rheumatol.* **17**, 885–7.

Taylor J, Mactier RA, Stewart WK *et al.* (1990). Effect of erythropoietin on anaemia in patients with myeloma receiving haemodialysis. *Br Med J.* **301**, 476–7.

US Recombinant Human Erythropoietin Predialysis Study Group (1991). Double-blind, placebo-controlled study of the therapeutic use of recombinant human erythropoietin for anemia associated with chronic renal failure in predialysis patients. *Am J Kid Dis.* **18**, 50–9.

van Wyck DB, Stivelman JC, Ruiz J *et al.* (1989). Iron status in patients receiving erythropoietin for dialysis- associated anemia. *Kidney International.* **35**, 712–16.

Vreugdenhil G, Wognum AW, van Eijk HG *et al.* (1990). Anaemia in rheumatoid arthritis: The role of iron, vitamin B_{12}, and folic acid deficiency, and erythropoietin responsiveness. *Ann Rheum Dis.* **49**, 93–8.

Walle AJ, Wong GY, Clemons GK *et al.* (1987). Erythropoietin-hematocrit feedback circuit in the anemia of end-stage renal disease. *Kid Intl.* **31**, 1205–9.

Winearls CG, Oliver DO, Pippard MJ *et al.* (1986). Effect of human erythropoietin derived from recombinant DNA on the anaemia of patients maintained by chronic haemodialysis. *Lancet.* **2**, 1175–1178.

Winearls CG, Sundal E, Stocker H *et al.* (1991). Recombinant human erythropoietin (epoetin alfa and beta) in patients on hemodialysis: Western Europe. In *Erythropoietin, molecular, cellular, and clinical biology*, ed. AJ Erslev, JW Adamson, JW Eschbach and CG Winearls, 291–318. Baltimore: The Johns Hopkins University Press.

Zachée P, Boogaerts MA, Lins RL *et al.* (1990). Erythropoietin, aluminium, and anaemia in patients on haemodialysis. *Lancet.* **335**, 1038–9.

3

GRANULOCYTE–MACROPHAGE COLONY-STIMULATING FACTOR

A. KHWAJA and D. C. LINCH

INTRODUCTION

Granulocyte–macrophage colony-stimulating factor (GM-CSF) was one of the first haemopoietic growth factors to be purified by painstaking biochemical separation techniques, but only minute quantities of protein were obtained (Gasson *et al.*, 1984). The cloning of the gene and the subsequent large-scale production of recombinant material enabled animal experiments and human trials to be carried out, culminating in the licensing of this product in the USA by the end of 1990. This astonishingly rapid development of a therapeutic agent reflects the interest in, and potential clinical importance of, the haemopoietic growth factors (HGFs).

BIOLOGY

Chromosomal location and protein structure

The gene for human GM-CSF has been mapped to the long arm of chromosome 5 (5q21–q32). This localization is interesting as the gene for interleukin-3 (IL-3) is only 9 kilobase pairs away and those for several other haemopoietic proteins, including macrophage colony-stimulating factor (M-CSF) and its receptor, IL-4 and IL-5 are also found on the long arm of chromosome 5 (van Leeuwen, 1989). Interstitial deletions in this region are common in myelodysplastic syndromes (MDS) and acute myeloid leukaemia (AML), especially when this is secondary to previous cytotoxic therapy (Nimer and Golde, 1987). Native GM-CSF has an apparent molecular weight between 15–32 kDa. This size variation is attributable to differing degrees of glycosylation (Clark and Kamen, 1987). Expression cloning of human GM-CSF shows that it is composed of 127 amino acid residues with approximately 50% sequence homology to murine GM-CSF but with no cross species reactivity (Wong *et al.*, 1985). Four cysteine residues form two intra-molecular disulphide bonds, which appear to be necessary for biological activity. Kaushansky *et al.* (1989) have utilized the lack of cross-reactivity between murine and human GM-CSF to construct hybrid molecules and have shown that two regions between amino acids 21 and 31, and 77 and 94 are likely to be involved in receptor binding.

Sites and regulation of production

GM-CSF is produced by a number of different cell types on appropriate activation. These include endothelial cells and fibroblasts exposed to tumour necrosis factor (TNF) or interleukin-1 (IL-1), macrophages stimulated by bacterial lipopolysaccharide (LPS) or adherence and T cells stimulated by antigen (Gasson, 1991). Thus, the homeostatic mechanisms involved in maintaining or increasing blood cell numbers may be intimately linked to the production of appropriate stimulatory cytokines by mature blood cells themselves, producing a system with multiple, complex cellular interactions. The presence of GM-CSF in synovial fluid from inflammatory arthropathies suggests that it may also play a part in mediating autoimmune responses (Williamson *et al.*, 1988).

Regulation of GM-CSF production at the cellular level involves a combination of both transcriptional and post-transcriptional control mechanisms (Devalia and Linch, 1991). The GM-CSF gene is constitutively transcribed in endothelial cells, monocytes and fibroblasts but accumulation of mRNA only occurs after cellular activation. This has been shown to be due to increased transcription and to stabilization of mRNA and various putative positive and negative regulatory elements have been described in the 3' untranslated region of the gene (Gasson, 1991). There is some debate as to the role of autocrine GM-CSF mRNA expression in acute myeloid leukaemia cells, which often bear surface receptors for GM-CSF and in some cases can proliferate in response to exogenous growth factor (Hoang *et al.*, 1986). The presence of GM-CSF mRNA in AML blasts can depend on the mode of cell preparation, as cells may become activated in vitro by purification steps, e.g. adherence (Gasson, 1991); some workers have suggested that other cytokines may be involved in inducing secondary GM-CSF production including via the endogenous secretion of IL-1 (Bradbury *et al.*, 1990).

A. KHWAJA & D. C. LINCH

Role in haemopoiesis

In vitro assays show that GM-CSF increases the production of neutrophil, eosinophil and monocyte colonies and under certain conditions will promote the formation of erythroid and megakaryocyte precursors (Clark and Kamen, 1987). GM-CSF is thought to act at the intermediate progenitor level and shows synergistic activity with early acting factors, e.g. stem cell factor (SCF) (Bernstein et al., 1991), other intermediate acting factors, e.g. IL-3 (Sieff et al., 1989), and with late acting factors, e.g. erythropoietin (EPO) (Sieff et al., 1985). Low concentrations of GM-CSF act preferentially on a common bipotential precursor to produce monocyte colonies and higher concentrations lead to the development of increased numbers of neutrophil colonies (Metcalf, 1985). GM-CSF is not normally detectable in the circulation and probably exerts its effects locally in a paracrine fashion. In support of this locally acting hypothesis, GM-CSF has been shown to bind to stromal elements in long-term bone marrow cultures (Gordon et al., 1987). The clinical administration of GM-CSF leads to striking increases in neutrophil, eosinophil and monocyte numbers, with a lesser effect on lymphocyte counts (Ganser et al., 1989). The last may be due to an increase in the production of other cytokines by accessory cells primed by GM-CSF and illustrates the complex haemopoietic responses that may be seen in vivo. GM-CSF administration also leads to marked increases in circulating myeloid and erythroid progenitor cells and this property has been utilized to increase the yield from leucapheresis in patients undergoing autologous peripheral blood progenitor cell transplants (Gianni et al., 1989).

Effects on mature cells

The availability of significant amounts of purified material led to the surprising observation that, in addition to its effects on haemopoietic progenitors, GM-CSF could alter the functional capabilities of neutrophils, eosinophils and monocyte/macrophages (Gasson et al., 1984). Such effects include enhanced survival, increased adhesion molecule expression, inhibition of migration, priming of the respiratory burst, enhanced direct and antibody-dependent cell mediated cytotoxicity (ADCC), increased microbial phagocytosis/killing, secretion of secondary granules and enhanced cytokine secretion.

GM-CSF may exert its effects directly, e.g. by increasing cellular adhesion molecule expression (Arnaout et al., 1992), or it may enhance the cell's responses to subsequent stimuli, e.g. by priming the neutrophil respiratory burst (Clark and Kamen, 1987). In a manner similar to that seen in haemopoiesis, GM-CSF can interact with other cytokines in activating neutrophil function. We have shown that GM-CSF and tumour necrosis factor alpha (TNFα) are highly synergistic in their effects on priming the neutrophil respiratory burst (Khwaja et al., 1992). Interestingly, no synergy was seen between GM-CSF and G-CSF, suggesting that in neutrophils these factors may either act on a similar responsive cell population or that they share a common post-receptor activation pathway. Therefore, the presence of low concentrations of GM-CSF at sites of inflammation/infection, either administered exogenously or produced locally by activated endothelial cells and monocyte/macrophages, may act to enhance host defence or mediate autoimmune responses. This enhancement of phagocyte function with GM-CSF treatment is potentially of value in the therapy of severe infection, in particular in the immune compromised patient.

Receptor and signal transduction

Cells responding to GM-CSF have relatively low numbers of specific surface receptors which exist in both low (K_d ~1 nM) and high (K_d ~50 pM) affinity forms. The structure of the GM-CSF receptor (GM-CSFR) has recently been elucidated and has been shown to belong to the haematopoietin receptor family that includes the receptors for EPO, IL-3, IL-4, IL-6, G-CSF and to show homology to certain non-haemopoietic receptors such as those for prolactin and growth hormone. The GM-CSF binding α chain is a transmembrane protein which when present on its own binds ligand with low affinity (Gearing et al., 1989). The association of this protein with a non-ligand binding β subunit comprises the high affinity GM-CSF receptor (Hayashida et al., 1990). There is evidence to suggest that this β subunit is shared with the IL-3R, as the addition of excess IL-3 to cells with both GM-CSF and IL-3 receptors inhibits total GM-CSF binding (Gesner et al., 1989). In this situation, only low affinity GM-CSF binding is detected in cells with both high and low affinity receptors (personal observation), presumably by utilization of the shared receptor component by the excess IL-3. With the data available to date, it is not clear if both subunits are required for signal transduction (Metcalf et al., 1990). Binding of GM-CSF to its receptor is followed by rapid ligand internalization, a process that may be phosphorylation-sensitive, and subsequent degradation; this step appears to down-regulate the cell's response to GM-CSF (Khwaja et al., 1990).

Intracellular mechanisms of GM-CSF signalling that follow ligand binding are not well understood. The GM-CSFR has no intrinsic tyrosine kinase activity, although rapid tyrosine and serine phosphorylation of unknown substrates has been described (Linnekin and Farrar, 1990). As with IL-3, GM-CSF has been shown to cause phosphorylation and activation of the c-*raf* protein at both serine and tyrosine residues (Carroll *et al.*, 1990). This proto-oncogene product is a cytosolic serine/threonine protein kinase and its rapid activation following GM-CSF binding suggests that it may be involved in transmitting mitogenic or other stimuli from the receptor to the interior of the cell. Although the GM-CSFR does not have the structure classically associated with G protein-mediated signalling, there are data to show that pretreatment with pertussis toxin, which inhibits many G proteins, can block some of the effects of GM-CSF (Gomez-Cambronero *et al.*, 1989). There is no consistent evidence for the activation of protein kinase C (PKC) by GM-CSF in neutrophils (Sullivan *et al.*, 1987) but PKC may be involved in mediating some of the effects of GM-CSF on more primitive cells (Adunyah *et al.*, 1991). Both leukotriene B_4 and platelet activating factor have been invoked as possible intermediaries in GM-CSF signalling and stimulation of macrophage proliferation by GM-CSF may be related to persistent activation of the Na^+/H^+ antiport (Gasson, 1991).

CLINICAL USES

Conventional chemotherapy

There are two main ways in which the use of GM-CSF in association with conventional dose chemotherapy may be of value. First, it may ameliorate myelotoxicity and thereby reduce infective morbidity; secondly, it may allow increases in delivered cytotoxic drug dose intensity. If the latter could be achieved, it would help to assess whether such increases translate into improved remission and survival rates in chemosensitive malignancies. Due to the wide variations in haematological toxicity of different chemotherapy regimens it may be difficult to extrapolate the results from any one study to a different treatment protocol. Several pilot studies of GM-CSF in this setting have been reported. These are, in the main, non-randomized trials with small numbers of patients, sometimes with many different diseases and treatment regimens within a single study.

The majority of trials have shown reductions in the depth and length of neutrophil nadirs with GM-CSF treatment. Two studies have compared haematological toxicity and infective morbidity between cycles of chemotherapy with and without GM-CSF in patients with solid tumours (Antman *et al.*, 1988; Herrmann *et al.*, 1990). There were reductions in neutropenia in both studies and Herrmann was able to show a reduction in the use of parenteral antibiotics and in days in hospital with GM-CSF; however, the effect of GM-CSF was less striking if the three patients undergoing double autologous bone marrow transplantation (ABMT) are excluded from analysis. More recently, Kaplan *et al.* (1991) have shown in a randomized trial after CHOP chemotherapy for HIV-associated NHL, that the administration of GM-CSF ameliorated neutropenia, reduced the admission rates for fever and allowed delivery of chemotherapy on schedule. The majority of patients receiving growth factor had stimulation of serum HIV-1 p24 antigen levels and there was no significant difference between GM-CSF patients and controls with regard to complete remission (CR) rates or overall survival.

Several investigators have reported that treatment with GM-CSF may reduce the depth of chemotherapy induced thrombocytopenia (DeVries *et al.*, 1991; Furman *et al.*, 1991). Data from Edmonson *et al.* (1989) suggest that this effect may be GM-CSF dose- and/or schedule-dependent: although the numbers involved are small, they were unable to show a beneficial effect at 10 µg/kg/day s.c. but could do so at 20 µg/kg/day, with the most marked effect seen with 12-hourly divided doses. In these studies, not all reductions in thrombocytopenia were clinically relevant and the beneficial effect of GM-CSF remains to be confirmed in randomized trials.

As the incidence of febrile neutropenia may be relatively low with many chemotherapy protocols, a more cost-effective way of using GM-CSF would be to not use it prophylactically in all patients but to start it in combination with antibiotics to treat fever as it occurs. Such a study has been carried out by Biesma, who randomized 30 patients receiving chemotherapy for a number of indications, predominantly breast and small-cell lung carcinoma, to receive GM-CSF or placebo at the onset of fever with leucopenia (mean absolute neutrophil count (ANC) was $< 0.1 \times 10^9/l$) (Biesma *et al.*, 1990). Although recovery neutrophil counts were higher in the GM-CSF-treated group, this effect was not clinically significant with no reduction in the number of days with fever or in the period of antibiotic administration. Another interesting study compared the effectiveness of GM-CSF with prophylactic antibiotics in reducing infective morbidity in patients receiving chemotherapy for recurrent lymphoma (Rodriguez *et al.*, 1990). Patients were randomized to receive either GM-CSF or oral ciprofloxacin and ketoconazole. GM-CSF-treated patients had a faster neutrophil recovery but required significantly more platelet and red cell transfusions. In addition, there were 12 documented infections over 27 chemotherapy cycles in the GM-CSF arm compared with 3 episodes over 24 cycles in the prophylactic antibiotic group. Because of these differences in clinical outcome, the study was stopped early.

In conclusion, the use of GM-CSF in association with conventional doses of chemotherapy cannot at present be recommended outside randomized trials. Trials should be designed to answer clinical questions and should be large and homogeneous enough in their patient population to stand a chance of doing so. Although data from several studies have suggested that GM-CSF administration can increase the proportion of patients who receive their chemotherapy at full doses on schedule, randomized studies are needed to show whether the consequent modest increases in dose intensity have any impact on tumour response rates. It is likely that further increases in chemotherapy doses will lead to more significant thrombocytopenia and to increased toxicity to organs other than the bone marrow.

Bone marrow transplantation

What can we hope to gain from the use of HGFs in bone marrow transplantation (BMT)? Shortening the period of post-BMT aplasia does not necessarily equate with improved survival. We have analysed early (before day +90 following BMT) mortality in 164 consecutive patients with Hodgkin's Disease (HD) undergoing autologous BMT (ABMT) following a chemotherapy based conditioning regimen. The data are shown in Table 3.1.

There was a total of 16 deaths, giving a treatment-related mortality of 9.75%. Eight deaths were of complications arising from non-marrow toxicity, four deaths occurred before day +14 during the period of complete aplasia which, as we will see from the published data, is unaffected by conventional treatment with GM-CSF, and three deaths were in patients with extensive Hodgkin's disease at post-mortem. Therefore, from these data at least, the scope for reduction in early deaths by the use of HGFs following ABMT is small and to detect an improvement with GM-CSF treatment would require a randomized trial with at least several hundreds of patients in each arm. In practice, any demonstrable benefit is likely to be restricted to decreased morbidity from infection and requirements for blood product support, with potential reductions in both the personal and financial costs associated with BMT.

Early dose-ranging phase I/II studies with GM-CSF were carried out by several investigators (Brandt et al., 1988; Nemunaitis et al., 1988; Devereux et al., 1989; Blazar et al., 1989) and the results of trials carried out in lymphoid malignancy are summarized in Table 3.2.

Table 3.1. *Causes of early (before day +90) mortality following autologous BMT for Hodgkin's Disease in 164 consecutive patients*

Day of death (post-ABMT)	Cause of death	Aetiology
6	Toxic colitis	Chemotherapy
7	Toxic colitis	Chemotherapy
8	Pseudomonas	Neutropenia
10	Fungal pneumonia	Neutropenia
14	*E. coli* septicaemia/ARDS	Neutropenia
14	Fungal pneumonia	Neutropenia
18	Fungal pneumonia	Neutropenia
18	*S. mitis* septicaemia/ARDS	Neutropenia + prog. HD
21	Progressive HD/colitis	Neutropenia + prog. HD
22	Idiopathic pneumonitis	Neutropenia + prog. HD
32	Bowel infarction	Chemotherapy
33	Interstitial pneumonitis	Chemotherapy
34	Interstitial pneumonitis	Chemotherapy
36	GVHD	Blood products
43	GVHD	Blood products
45	Interstitial pneumonitis	Chemotherapy

prog. HD, progressive Hodgkin's disease.

With the exception of the trial conducted by Blazar, all the trials showed accelerated neutrophil recovery when treated patients were compared with historical controls. This trial differed from others in the use of in vitro marrow purging with 4-hydroperoxycyclophosphamide. Patients receiving > 1.2×10^4 CFU-GM/kg had accelerated neutrophil recovery when compared with patients receiving less than this figure – unfortunately, comparable data for control patients matched for CFU numbers were not provided, making it difficult to ascertain whether GM-CSF treatment had any significant effects in this setting. None of the phase I/II trials showed any clear improvement in platelet recovery following BMT. The trial by Nemunaitis *et al.* has been interpreted as showing accelerated platelet recovery with GM-CSF treatment at doses between 60 and 240 $\mu g/m^2$ (Nemunaitis *et al.*, 1988). However, comparison was made with a large number of historical controls and changes in transplant practice may have influenced haematological recovery. It is

Table 3.2. *Phase I/II trials of GM-CSF in autologous BMT for lymphoid malignancy*

	Days to ANC > 500 ×10⁶/l	Days to platelet independ- ence	Days to plat. > 50 x 10⁹/l	Days of fever	Days in hospital	Number of patients	Reference
GM-CSF							Nemunaitis
< 60 mcg	22	30	NA	11	30	6	(1988)
> 60 mcg	14	29	NA	6	29	8	
Controls	25	38	NA	12	41	86	
GM-CSF	16*	NA	30	5	30	12	Devereux
							(1989)
Controls	25	NA	28	5	30	19	
GM-CSF		Plat.units					Blazar
<60 mcg	23	92	NA	NA	NA	5	(1989)
>60 mcg	23	156	NA	NA	NA	16	
Controls	24	149	NA	NA	NA	27	

* Statistically significant difference from controls; NA, not applicable; Plat. units, platelet units transfused.

interesting to note that concurrent patients receiving < 60 μg/m² GM-CSF, who did not have accelerated neutrophil recovery when compared to historical controls, had similar platelet requirements and hospital stay to the higher dose GM-CSF group. The effects of GM-CSF treatment on measures of morbidity were inconsistent in these early studies and do not allow any firm conclusions to be made as to its clinical efficacy.

Therefore, the data from the phase I/II trials confirmed the in vitro and pre-clinical animal studies of the effects of GM-CSF on the generation of mature myeloid cells, but did not demonstrate any significant biological activity on platelet or red cell production. Recently, several randomized trials of GM-CSF in autologous BMT have been reported (Nemunaitis *et al.*, 1991a; BNLI, 1991) and the results are summarized in Table 3.3. All trials confirm that GM-CSF at a dose of 250 μg/m²/day reduces the period of neutropenia following BMT. However, where the data were given, no reduction was seen in the period of absolute neutropaenia (ANC $< 0.1 \times 10^9$/l), the time of maximum risk of infection. Despite striking reductions of at least 7 days in the neutropenic phase (ANC $< 0.5 \times 10^9$/l) in each study, the number of febrile days were similar in both treated and control patients, and there were only small or no reductions seen in the number of days on antibiotics or antifungals. It has been our experience with GM-CSF-treated patients that clinical improvement does not always parallel neutrophil recovery. This may be attributable to the known side-effects of GM-CSF, which include fever (see below).

No improvement in platelet recovery was seen in any of the trials, with two studies showing a trend towards prolonged platelet dependence in the GM-CSF arm. However, two of the four studies showed a significant reduction in the period of hospitalization following BMT. Toxicity due to GM-CSF during the transplant phase was minor but the US trial is the only one for which survival data are available. This study showed eight early deaths (before day 100) in both arms of the trial and no adverse effect of GM-CSF on early rates of relapse in patients with lymphoid neoplasia.

In addition to the trials in autologous BMT, there have been two reported trials of GM-CSF in allogeneic (allo) BMT (Nemunaitis *et al.*, 1991b; Powles *et al.*, 1991). Nemunaitis *et al.* performed a phase I/II study in 47 patients undergoing alloBMT for a variety of indications; good risk patients with myeloid malignancy were excluded. This study showed that GM-CSF treatment did not affect neutrophil recovery to 0.1×10^9/l but did accelerate recovery to 1.0×10^9/l by 4-5 days at all doses between 30 and 500 μg/m^2. No effect on platelet recovery was seen and there was no significant difference in length of hospitalization. 100-day mortality was 28%, 2 of 12 patients transplanted for myeloid malignancy relapsed before day 100, and no adverse effect on incidence or severity of graft-versus-host disease (GVHD) was seen. In a controlled trial, Powles *et al.* randomized 40 patients with acute and chronic leukaemia, the majority myeloid, to placebo or GM-CSF at 8 μg/kg/day for 14 days. This trial showed a statistically non-significant reduction in the time taken to reach an ANC of 0.5×10^9/l in the GM-CSF treated group (13 versus 16 days). However, patients receiving GM-CSF required significantly more antibiotics, had lower platelet counts between days 7 and 14, an increased requirement for red cell transfusion, and significant increases in blood urea, creatinine and bilirubin concentrations at day 14. There was no adverse effect of GM-CSF on the incidence and grade of GVHD and hospital stay was the same in both groups. No increase in relapse rates was seen in the GM-CSF-treated arm.

Table 3.3. *Randomized trials of GM-CSF in autologous BMT for lymphoid malignancy*

	Days to ANC > 500 × 10⁶/l	Days to platelet independence	Days of fever	Days on antibiotic	Days in hospital	Number of patients	Reference
GM-CSF	19*	26	8	24*	27*	65	Nemunaitis
Placebo	26	29	8	27	33	63	(1991a)
GM-CSF	15*	39	NA	19	30	39	Link
Placebo	28	31	NA	19	31	40	(1990)
GM-CSF	14*	19	4	19	23*	41	Gorin
Placebo	21	19	2	22	28	47	(1990)
GM-CSF	14*	25	7	11	24	26	BNLI
Placebo	22	19	6	10	25	28	(1991)

* Statistically significant difference from controls; NA, not applicable.

Recently, there has been increasing interest in the use of high dose cytotoxic therapy combined with haematological rescue with peripheral blood progenitor cells (PBPC) instead of, or in addition to, autologous bone marrow. The ability of GM-CSF to expand the PBPC compartment has been utilized in several pilot studies. Gianni *et al.* (1989) treated seven patients with lymphoma with high-dose cyclophosphamide and GM-CSF followed by 3–4 leucaphereses in the recovery phase from the cyclophosphamide induced aplasia. Patients were then conditioned with melphalan/total body irradiation (TBI) and received both autologous marrow and PBPC. Comparison was made with a control group who were leucapheresed after cyclophosphamide alone. In addition, four of the seven patients received GM-CSF after transplant. Neutrophil recovery to $0.5 \times 10^9/l$ was short in both groups (9 and 11 days) and platelet recovery to $50 \times 10^9/l$ was 11 days and 17 days in the GM-CSF group and controls respectively. Neutrophil counts of less than $0.1 \times 10^9/l$ were only seen for 1–3 days in the GM-CSF primed group. Spitzer (1991) conducted a trial of chemotherapy/GM-CSF-mobilized PBPC where patients initially underwent a bone marrow harvest divided into two aliquots. In cycle 1 patients were given GM-CSF after marrow infusion alone (the conditioning regimen was Cyclo/VP-16/cisplatinum) and in cycle 2 they were also given PBPC. There was no effect of PBPC on early neutrophil recovery to $0.1 \times 10^9/l$ or on fever/infection, but there was a significant reduction in thrombocytopenia. It is apparent that transplantation with PBPC requires considerable organizational and financial effort, and the role of CSFs therein remains to be defined.

GM-CSF has also been employed for delayed engraftment following BMT. Responses are variable, but there is a suggestion that survival may be improved compared to historical controls, except in chemically purged ABMT (Nemunaitis et al., 1990; Branwein *et al.*, 1991).

In conclusion, it is still not clear whether the use of GM-CSF in BMT is justifiable on a routine basis. The conflicting data in the ABMT trials may, to some degree, be due to the heterogeneous mix of diseases and remission states and to the lack of uniformity in conditioning protocols within individual trials. Although GM-CSF has reduced the length of the neutropenic phase in each trial, this has not consistently translated into an improvement for the patient or a reduction in the financial costs of treatment. Different BMT protocols may need to be assessed individually to ascertain whether treatment with single agent GM-CSF is clinically beneficial. At present, the use of GM-CSF in the treatment of good risk patients undergoing BMT for myeloid malignancies is not justifiable as the risk of stimulating the survival and/or growth of residual leukaemic cells outweighs any potential benefits. Treatment of poor risk patients with myeloid leukaemia with GM-CSF should be confined to the trial setting.

Aplastic anaemia

There have been several small studies examining the short-term effects of GM-CSF in aplastic anaemia (Antin *et al.*, 1988; Vadhan-Raj *et al.*, 1988; Champlin *et al.*, 1989; Guinan *et al.*, 1990). The overall impression in adult patients is that GM-CSF may increase neutrophil counts significantly in some patients, but these are likely to be those with detectable residual myelopoiesis and higher pretreatment neutrophil numbers. No consistent effect on platelet or red cell requirements has been seen. The responses in children have been more encouraging but the data are still inconclusive as to the true value of treatment (Guinan *et al.*, 1990). Patients treated with GM-CSF may have an increased risk of alloimmunization via exposure to blood products and treatment should not be given lightly to those patients likely to undergo subsequent BMT. There may be a role for growth factor treatment in patients for whom BMT is not an option, perhaps in conjunction with, or following, immunosuppressive treatment. It is likely that in the future combination HGF therapy will be more useful in such a setting; for the present in view of the lack of a multilineage effect, it is not clear if treatment with GM-CSF offers any significant advantage over G-CSF, which has a lower incidence of side-effects.

Congenital neutropenia

This term describes a heterogeneous collection of disorders characterized by varying levels of neutropenia with a similarly broad range of clinical features. The administration of GM-CSF to five patients with severe congenital neutropenia (Kostmann syndrome) led to an increase in mature neutrophil numbers in only one and had a marked dose-dependent effect on eosinophil production in the other four (Welte et al., 1990). Despite the lack of effect of GM-CSF on increasing the neutrophil count there were some clinical responses with resolution of gingivostomatitis and a reduction in new episodes of severe bacterial infection; these were presumably attributable to the eosinophilia. The poor neutrophil response to GM-CSF contrasted with significant increases seen following later G-CSF treatment. These have been maintained over long periods and shown to be of marked clinical benefit (Bonilla et al., 1989). Similar results have been obtained in the treatment of cyclic neutropenia (Hammond et al., 1989). Therefore, there is a considerable body of experience with long-term administration of G-CSF in the congenital neutropenias and this has been shown to be both effective and safe. At the present time G-CSF must be regarded as the treatment of choice for these rare disorders.

Myelodysplasia/acute myeloid leukaemia

GM-CSF has been used in the treatment of myeloid malignancies with several aims in mind. First, to try and ameliorate the pancytopenia of MDS thereby reducing the risk of infection and the requirement for blood product support. Secondly, the presence of functional GM-CSF receptors on leukaemic blasts has been exploited to try and recruit quiescent cells into the cell cycle and then to administer cycle-specific cytotoxic therapy. Finally, several investigators have used GM-CSF to stimulate haematological recovery following induction chemotherapy, in particular in patients at a high risk of death from infection in the aplastic phase.

Treatment of MDS with GM-CSF has consistently led to increases in neutrophil and eosinophil granulocytes in the majority of patients (Vadhan-Raj et al., 1987; Antin et al., 1988; Ganser et al., 1989; Thompson et al.,

1989; Rosenfeld *et al.*, 1991). Although increases in reticulocytes have been seen in a significant proportion of patients, this has rarely translated into a reduction in transfusion requirements. Disappointingly, platelet responses have been infrequent and significant reductions in platelet numbers have also been reported (Dunbar *et al.*, 1990). In the trial carried out by Thompson, initial treatment with GM-CSF was associated with an increase in neutrophil numbers. However, after 1–2 weeks treatment, there was then a reduction in neutrophil counts, in some cases to pretreatment levels of severe neutropenia. This was associated with the development of neutralizing antibodies in at least one patient and antibodies have also been reported with prolonged treatment in another trial (Dunbar *et al.*, 1990). There may be an increased risk of transformation to AML in patients with high pretreatment blast counts (Ganser *et al.*, 1989) and GM-CSF should probably not be administered on its own to patients with bone marrow blasts greater than 10%.

In vitro studies have shown that GM-CSF can increase the percentage of AML blasts that are actively cycling and that follow-up treatment with cycle-specific cytotoxics can increase cell kill (Bhalia *et al.*, 1988). This approach has also been adopted in vivo in both high and low risk patients. Bettelheim *et al.* (1991) treated 18 patients with de novo AML with GM-CSF 24–48 h before chemotherapy and continued it until neutrophil recovery had occurred. They were able to show recruitment of blasts into drug-sensitive phases of the cell cycle and increases in prechemotherapy blast numbers. Neutrophil recovery was accelerated compared to historical controls, with no effect on platelet regeneration, and the overall CR rate was 83%. Two studies of GM-CSF following chemotherapy for patients with poor risk AML have shown conflicting results, with one centre reporting accelerated neutrophil recovery and another no impact on either neutrophil regeneration or infective deaths (Buechner *et al.*, 1990; Estey *et al.*, 1990). Leukaemic regrowth during GM-CSF treatment was observed in several patients and was reversible in one patient on stopping the growth factor. No conclusions can be reached about long-term remission or survival from these studies. The confirmation that GM-CSF can stimulate the cycling and growth of myeloid blasts in vivo has implications for its use in reducing morbidity and mortality in good risk patients with AML. With the high CR rates currently obtainable in such patients with standard therapy, there may be little to gain by the use of growth factors with a significant theoretical risk of enhancing leukaemic regrowth.

Activation of phagocyte function

We and others have shown that many of the in vitro effects of GM-CSF on enhancing the functional capabilities of neutrophils and monocyte/macrophages can also be demonstrated in vivo in patients receiving GM-CSF treatment (Khwaja *et al.*, 1992). The ability to enhance certain phagocyte functions, such as microbial ingestion and killing and tumour cytotoxicity, raises the possibility of using GM-CSF as adjunctive anti-infection or antitumour therapy. GM-CSF has been shown to protect mice from death from experimentally induced bacterial infection if treatment is started within 1–2 days of microbial exposure (Morrissey and Charrier, 1990). Of some concern are the possible detrimental effects of GM-CSF on host defence following inhibition of neutrophil migration. Cioffi *et al.* (1991) have recently described two abscesses requiring surgical drainage in a group of ten burns patients receiving GM-CSF. There is also a significant risk of pulmonary toxicity in patients with relatively high leucocyte counts and GM-CSF may lead to the worsening of pre-existing lung injury or infection (Devereux *et al.*, 1989; Cioffi *et al.*, 1991). It is possible that low doses of GM-CSF will have a beneficial effect on phagocyte function with a reduced risk of toxicity but it may prove difficult to design a study to convincingly demonstrate a clinical advantage.

Pharmacology and toxicity

Recombinant GM-CSF has been synthesized in bacterial (non-glycosylated), yeast and mammalian (both glycosylated) cell systems and studies have been reported using each of these products. It is not clear whether there are any clinically significant differences between these forms but in vitro studies show that increasing glycosylation of native lymphocyte-derived GM-CSF leads to a reduction in receptor affinity (Cebon *et al.*, 1990a). In vivo studies have suggested that the more heavily glycosylated forms are cleared relatively slowly but the practical consequences of this phenomenon are not known (Clark & Kamen 1987). GM-CSF may be given by the intravenous or subcutaneous routes. Intravenous bolus administration leads to rapid high peak serum levels which are associated with an increased likelihood of side-effects; there is a biphasic clearance curve with a dose-dependent terminal half-life of 30–60 min. Subcutaneous bolus injection is associated with a delayed peak concentration (~ 4 h) and the greatest area under the concentration–time curve (Cebon *et al.*, 1990b). Prolonged

Table 3.4. *Reported side-effects of treatment with GM-CSF*

High doses only (> ~ 20 µg/kg)	Capillary leak syndrome, central vein central vein thrombosis, hypotension
Seen over a wide dose range	Fever, pleuritis, myalgia, pulmonary infiltrates, bone pain, hypoxia (first-dose effect), phlebitis, splenomegaly, skin rash, hypoalbuminaemia, pericarditis, increased LDH/alkaline phosphatase, thrombocytopenia (relapse of ITP)

ITP, idiopathic thrombocytopenic purpura.

therapeutic levels can also be obtained by continuous i.v. infusion. Only a minute proportion of the total dose given appears as immunoreactive GM-CSF in the urine and clearance may be mediated by target cells as is the case for M-CSF and G-CSF (Layton *et al.*, 1989). Effective doses vary between the patient populations being treated. In autologous BMT, therapeutic effects have mainly been seen in patients receiving the equivalent of 60–250 µg/m²/day but lower doses may be effective in other conditions.

GM-CSF toxicity can be divided into that which is seen at most doses, e.g. fever and bone pain, and those effects seen only at very high doses, e.g. central vein thrombosis. These higher doses have now been shown to be therapeutically unnecessary. Table 3.4 lists these toxicities. A first-dose effect of flushing, tachycardia, hypotension and hypoxia has been described by Lieschke *et al.* (1989a) and was found to be more common in patients receiving GM-CSF intravenously rather than subcutaneously, especially at doses above 3 µg/kg. Patients with very high granulocyte counts, in particular eosinophils, are more likely to suffer pulmonary toxicity with the development of infiltrates (Nissen *et al.*, 1988). This may be related to the margination of neutrophils and monocytes in the lung within 15 minutes of starting intravenous GM-CSF (Devereux *et al.*, 1987) and treatment with this growth factor should probably be withheld from patients with large numbers of circulating granulocytes. It has also been our experience that side-effects such as fever and malaise are more frequent when the white cell count is still relatively normal, usually in the period prior to the nadir that follows cytotoxic therapy. Transient splenomegaly may develop during treatment and can give rise to fears of relapse in patients with lymphoid neoplasia (personal observation). Reductions in serum cholesterol and albumin are probably due to a temporary impairment of hepatic biosynthesis and levels return to normal once treatment is stopped (Takahashi et al., 1991).

A fall in platelet numbers has been shown to occur with treatment of haematologically normal patients over a period of days (Herrmann et al., 1990) and a relapse of previous auto-immune thrombocytopenia has also been reported (Lieschke et al., 1989b). These platelet changes probably reflect activation of the reticuloendothelial system and have also been described in patients receiving M-CSF and G-CSF (Khwaja et al., 1991). Due to the propensity of GM-CSF to cause phlebitis its intravenous administration should be into a large central vein. The ease of subcutaneous delivery with the achievement of sustained therapeutic serum levels has meant that this has often been the route of choice, especially in outpatient-based protocols. Injections by this route can cause local stinging that lasts for 10–15 min and may occasionally lead to the development of a skin infiltrate, with a local predominance of perivascular lymphocytes and eosinophils (De Vries et al., 1991). Although the list of potential side-effects appears formidable, having to stop GM-CSF for reasons of toxicity is a relatively unusual occurrence in practice. The limited data available so far in the paediatric use of GM-CSF suggest that doses that cause significant toxicity in adults are well tolerated by children (Furman, 1991).

Patients undergoing ABMT may develop antibodies to recombinant GM-CSF produced in yeast and these are directed to epitopes that normally undergo O-linked glycosylation in the native form (Gribben et al., 1990). Others have also reported antibodies and these have been associated with loss of therapeutic effect in at least one case (Thompson et al., 1989). Although the relevance of these antibodies may be limited in the short-term use of GM-CSF, its effectiveness in prolonged or repeated use may be negated by antibody-mediated neutralization of biological activity or by enhanced clearance from the blood.

In addition to their presence on haemopoietic cells, receptors for GM-CSF have been demonstrated on numerous other cell types. These have been found on several malignant cell lines, including those derived from small-cell lung carcinoma, choriocarcinoma, colon adenocarcinoma and malignant melanoma and also on fresh biopsy specimens from various solid tumours (Gasson, 1991). The responses of these cells to GM-CSF are not predictable and its addition can cause growth stimulation, growth inhibition, or have no effect at all. The results of both pilot and randomized trials in lymphoid tumours have so far not shown any reduction in response rates or any increase in the incidence of relapse (Nemunaitis et al., 1991a,c). Future trials of GM-CSF should address this question directly in order to assess the relevance of in vitro findings to the clinical setting.

CONCLUSIONS

GM-CSF has been shown to have pronounced effects on primitive and mature myeloid cells both in vitro and in vivo. It is now licensed in the USA for the amelioration of neutropenia following bone marrow transplantation but its true clinical value in this and other settings has not as yet been fully elucidated. In the future, GM-CSF is likely to be used in combination with other haemopoietic growth factors in the hope of obtaining synergistic responses without increased toxicity.

REFERENCES

Adunyah SE, Unlap TM, Wagner F and Kraft AS (1991). Regulation of c-*jun* expression and AP-1 enhancer activity by GM-CSF. *J Biol Chem.* **266**, 5670–5.

Antin JH, Smith BR, Holmes W and Rosenthal DS (1988). Phase I/II study of recombinant human GM-CSF in aplastic anemia and myelodysplastic syndrome. *Blood.* **72**, 705–713.

Antman KS, Griffin JD, Elias A *et al.* (1988). Effect of recombinant human GM-CSF on chemotherapy induced myelosuppression. *N Engl J Med.* **319**, 593–8.

Arnaout MA, Wang EA, Clark SC and Sieff CA (1986). Human recombinant GM-CSF increases cell to cell adhesion and surface expression of adhesion promoting glycoproteins on mature granulocytes. *J Clin Invest.* **8**, 596–601.

Bernstein ID, Andrews RG and Zsebo KM (1991). Recombinant human stem cell factor enhances the formation of colonies by CD34+ and CD34+lin- cells, and the generation of colony forming cell progeny from CD34+lin- cells cultured with IL-3, G-CSF or GM-CSF. *Blood.* **77**, 2316–21.

Bettelheim P, Valent P, Andreef M *et al.* (1991). Recombinant human GM-CSF in combination with standard induction therapy in de novo acute myeloid leukaemia. *Blood.* **77**, 700–11.

Bhalia K, Birkhofer M, Arlin Z *et al.* (1988). Effect of recombinant GM-CSF on the metabolism of cytosine arabinoside in normal and leukemic human bone marrow cells. *Leukemia.* **2**, 810.

Biesma B, De Vries EGE, Willemse PHB *et al.* (1990). Efficacy and tolerability of recombinant human GM-CSF in patients with chemotherapy-related leukopenia and fever. *Eur J Cancer.* **26**, 932–6.

Blazar BR, Kersey JH, McGlave PB *et al.* (1989). In vivo administration of recombinant human GM-CSF in acute lymphoblastic leukemia patients receiving purged autografts. *Blood.* **73**, 849–57.

BNLI (British National Lymphoma Investigation) (1991). A randomised double-blind placebo-controlled trial of GM-CSF in lymphoma ABMT (in press).

Bonilla MA, Gillio AP, Ruggerio M *et al.* (1989). Effects of recombinant human G-CSF on neutropenia in patients with congenital agranulocytosis. *N Engl J Med.* **320**, 1574.

A. KHWAJA & D. C. LINCH

Bradbury D, Bowen G, Kozlowski R, Reilly I and Russell N (1990). Endogenous IL-1 can regulate the autonomous growth of the blast cells of acute myeloblastic leukaemia by inducing autocrine stimulation of GM-CSF. *Leukemia*. **4**, 44.

Brandt SJ, Peters WP, Atwater SK *et al.* (1988). Effect of recombinant human GM-CSF on haemopoietic reconstruction after high-dose chemotherapy and autologous bone marrow transplantation. *N Engl J Med*. **318**, 869-76.

Branwein JM, Nayar R, Baker MA *et al.* (1991). GM-CSF therapy for delayed engraftment after autologous BMT. *Exp Haematol*. **19**, 191–5.

Buechner T, Hiddemann W, Koenigsmann *et al.* (1990). Recombinant human GM-CSF following chemotherapy in high-risk AML. *Bone Marrow Transplant*. **6** (**Suppl.**), 131.

Carroll MP, Clark-Lewis I, Rapp UR and May WS (1990). IL-3 and GM-CSF mediate rapid phosphorylation and activation of cytosolic c-*raf*. *J Biol Chem* **265**, 19812–17.

Cebon J, Nicola N, Ward M *et al.* (1990a). GM-CSF from human lymphocytes. *J Biol Chem*. **265**, 4483–91.

Cebon JS, Bury RW, Lieschke GJ and Morstyn G (1990b). The effects of dose and route of administration on the pharmacokinetics of GM-CSF. *Eur J Cancer*. **26**, 1064–9.

Champlin RE, Nimer SD, Ireland P, Oette DH and Golde DW (1989). Treatment of refractory aplastic anemia with recombinant human GM-CSF. *Blood*. **73**, 694.

Cioffi WG, Burleson DG, Jordan BS *et al.* (1991). Effects of GM-CSF in burns patients. *Arch Surg*. **126**, 74–9.

Clark SC, Kamen R (1987). The human hematopoietic colony-stimulating factors. *Science*. **236**, 1229–37.

De Vries EGE, Biesma B, Willemse PHB *et al.* (1991). A double-blind placebo-controlled study with GM-CSF during chemotherapy for ovarian cancer. *Cancer Res*. **51**, 116–22.

Devalia V and Linch DC (1991). Haemopoietic regulation by growth factors. *Cambridge Medical Reviews: Haematological Oncology*, Volume 1, 1–28. Cambridge University Press.

Devereux S, Linch DC, Campos-Costa D *et al.* (1987). Transient leucopenia induced by GM-CSF. *Lancet*. **ii**, 1523.

Devereux S, Linch DC, Gribben JG *et al.* (1989). GM-CSF accelerates neutrophil recovery after bone marrow transplantation for Hodgkin's disease. *Bone Marrow Transplantation*. **4**, 49–54.

Dunbar CE, Smith D, Kimball J, Garrison L, Nienhuis AW and Young NS (1990). Sequential treatment with recombinant human growth factors to compare activity of GM-CSF and IL3 in the treatment of primary myelodysplasia. *Blood*. **76** (**Suppl. 1**), 141a (abstract).

Edmondson JH, Long HJ, Jeffreis JA, Buckner JC, Colon-Otero G and Fitch TR (1989). Amelioration of chemotherapy-induced thrombocytopenia by GM-CSF: apparent dose and schedule dependency. *J Natl Cancer Inst.* **81**, 1510–12 (letter).

Estey EH, Dixon D, Kantarjian HM *et al.* (1990). Treatment of poor-prognosis newly diagnosed AML with Ara-C and recombinant human GM-CSF. *Blood.* **75**, 1766.

Furman WL, Fairclough DL, Huhn RD *et al.* (1991). Therapeutic effects and pharmacokinetics of recombinant human GM-CSF in childhood cancer patients receiving myelosuppressive chemotherapy. *J Clin Oncol.* **9**, 1022–8.

Ganser A, Volkers B, Greher J *et al.* (1989). Recombinant human GM-CSF in patients with myelodysplastic syndromes – a phase I/II trial. *Blood.* **73**, 31–7.

Gasson JC (1991). Molecular physiology of GM-CSF. *Blood.* **77**, 1131–45.

Gasson JC, Weisbart RH, Kaufman SE *et al.* (1984). Purified human GM-CSF: direct action on neutrophils. *Science.* **226**, 1339–42.

Gearing DP, King JA, Gough NM and Nicola NA (1989). Expression cloning of a receptor for human GM-CSF. *EMBO J.* **8**, 3667–76.

Gesner T, Mufson RA, Turner KJ and Clark SC (1989). Identification through chemical cross-linking of distinct GM-CSF and IL-3 receptors on myeloid leukemic cells, KG-1. *Blood.* **74**, 2652–56.

Gianni AM, Siena S, Bregni M *et al.* (1989). GM-CSF to harvest circulating stem cells for autotransplantation. *Lancet.* **ii**, 580–85.

Gomez-Cambronero J, Yamazaki M, Metwally F *et al.* (1989). GM-CSF and human neutrophils: role of guanine nucleotide regulatory proteins. *Proc Natl Acad Sci USA.* **86**, 3569–73.

Gordon MY, Riley GP, Watt SM and Greaves MF (1987). Compartmentalisation of a hemopoietic growth factor (GM-CSF) by glycosaminoglycans in the bone marrow microenvironment. *Nature.* **326**, 403–5.

Gribben JG, Devereux S, Thomas NSB *et al.* (1990). Development of antibodies to unprotected glycosylation sites on recombinant human GM-CSF. *Lancet.* **i**, 434–8.

Guinan EC, Sieff CA, Oette DH and Nathan DG (1990). A phase I/II trial of recombinant GM-CSF for children with aplastic anemia. *Blood.* **76**, 1077–82.

Hammond WP, Price TH, Souza LM and Dale DC (1989). Treatment of cyclic neutropenia with G-CSF. *N Engl J Med.* **320**, 1306.

Hayashida K, Kitamura T, Gorman DM, Arai K-I, Yokota T and Miyajima A (1990). Molecular cloning of a second subunit of the receptor for human GM-CSF: reconstitution of a high affinity GM-CSF receptor. *Proc Natl Acad Sci USA.* **87**, 9655–9.

Herrmann F, Sculz G, Wieser M *et al.* (1990). Effect of GM-CSF on neutropenia and related morbidity induced by myelotoxic chemotherapy. *Am J Med.* **88**, 619–24.

Hoang T, Nara N, Wong G *et al.* (1986). Effects of recombinant GM-CSF on the blast cells of acute myeloblastic leukemia. *Blood.* **68**, 313–16.

Kaplan LD, Kahn JO, Crowe S *et al.* (1991). Clinical and virologic effects of recombinant human GM-CSF in patients receiving chemotherapy for human immunodeficiency virus-associated non-Hodgkin's lymphoma: results of a randomized trial. *J Clin Oncol.* **9**, 929–40.

Kaushansky K, Shoemaker SG, Alfaro S and Brown C (1989). Hematopoietic activity of GM-CSF is dependent upon two distinct regions of the molecule: functional analysis based upon the activities of interspecies hybrid growth factors. *Proc Natl Acad Sci USA.* **86**, 1213.

Khwaja A, Roberts PJ, Jones HM, Yong K, Jaswon MS and Linch DC (1990). Isoquinolinesulfonamide protein kinase inhibitors H7 and H8 enhance the effects of GM-CSF on neutrophil function and inhibit GM-CSF receptor internalisation. *Blood.* **76**, 996–1003.

Khwaja A, Johnson B, Addison IE, Yong K, Ruthven K, Abramson S and Linch DC (1991). In vivo effects of macrophage colony-stimulating factor on human monocyte function. *Br J Haematol.* **77**, 25–31.

Khwaja A, Carver J and Linch DC (1992). The interaction of GM-CSF, G-CSF, and TNFα on the priming of the neutrophil respiratory burst. *Blood.* **79**, 145–53.

Layton JE, Hockman H and Morstyn G (1989). Evidence for a novel in vivo control mechanism of granulopoiesis: mature cell-related control of a regulatory growth factor. *Blood.* **74**, 1303–7.

Lieschke GJ, Cebon J and Morstyn G (1989a). Characterisation of the clinical effects after the first dose of bacterially synthesised recombinant human GM-CSF. *Blood.* **74**, 2634–43.

Lieschke GJ, Maher D, Cebon J *et al.* (1989b). Effects of subcutaneously administered bacterially-synthesized recombinant human GM-CSF in patients with advanced malignancy. *Ann Int Med.* **110**, 357–364.

Linnekin D and Farrar WL (1990). Signal transduction of human IL-3 and GM-CSF through serine and tyrosine phosphorylation. *Biochem J.* **271**, 317–24.

Metcalf D (1985). The granulocyte-macrophage colony-stimulating factors. *Science.* **229**, 16–22.

Metcalf D, Nicola NA, Gearing DP and Gough NM (1990). Low affinity placenta-derived receptors for human GM-CSF can deliver a proliferative signal to murine hematopoietic cells. *Proc Natl Acad Sci USA.* **87**, 4670–4.

Morrissey PJ and Charrier K (1990). GM-CSF administration augments the survival of ITY-resistant A/J mice, but not ITY-susceptible C57BL/6 mice, to a lethal challenge with salmonella typhimurium. *J Immunol.* **144**, 557–561.

Nemunaitis J, Singer JW, Buckner CD *et al.* (1988). Use of recombinant human GM-CSF in autologous BMT for lymphoid malignancies. *Blood.* **72**, 834–6.

Nemunaitis J, Singer JW, Buckner CD *et al.* (1990). Use of recombinant GM-CSF in graft failure after BMT. *Blood.* **76**, 245–53.

Nemunaitis J, Rabinowe SN, Singer JW *et al.* (1991a). Recombinant human GM-CSF after autologous BMT for lymphoid cancer. *N Engl J Med.* **324**, 1773–8.

GRANULOCYTE–MACROPHAGE COLONY-STIMULATING FACTOR

Nemunaitis J, Buckner CD, Appelbaum F *et al.* (1991b). Phase I/II trial of recombinant human GM-CSF following allogeneic bone marrow transplantation. *Blood.* **77**, 2065–71.

Nemunaitis J, Singer JW, Buckner CD *et al.* (1991c). Long-term follow-up of patients who received recombinant human GM-CSF after autologous bone marrow transplantation for lymphoid malignancy. *Bone Marrow Transplant.* **7**, 49–52.

Nimer SD and Golde DW (1987). The 5q- abnormality. *Blood.* **70**, 1705.

Nissen C, Tichelli A, Gratwohl A *et al.* (1988). Failure of GM-CSF therapy in aplastic anaemia patients with very severe neutropenia. *Blood.* **72**, 2045–51.

Powles R, Smith C, Milan S *et al.* (1991). Human recombinant GM-CSF in allogeneic bone marrow transplantation for leukaemia: double-blind, placebo-controlled trial. *Lancet.* **336**, 1417–20.

Rodriguez M, Swan F, Hagenmeister F *et al.* (1990). High dose ESHAP with GM-CSF vs. prophylactic antibiotics. *Blood.* **76 (Suppl. 1)**, 370a (abstract).

Rosenfeld CS, Sulecki M, Evans C and Sadduck RK (1991). Comparison of intravenous versus subcutaneous recombinant human GM-CSF in patients with primary myelodysplasia. *Exp Hematol.* **19**, 273–7.

Sieff CA, Emerson SG, Donahue RE *et al.* (1985). Human recombinant GM-CSF: a multilineage hematopoietin. *Science.* **230**, 1171.

Sieff CA, Ekern SC, Nathan DG and Anderson JW (1989). Combinations of recombinant colony-stimulating factors are required for optimal hematopoietic differentiation in serum-deprived culture. *Blood.* **73**, 688–93.

Spitzer G (1991). Autologous bone marrow transplantation in solid tumors. *Current Opinion in Oncology.* **3**, 238–44.

Sullivan R, Griffin JD, Simons ER *et al.* (1987). Effects of recombinant human GM-CSF on signal transduction pathways in human granulocytes. *J Immunol.* **139**, 3422–30.

Takahashi M, Nikkuni K, Moriyama Y and Shibata A (1991). GM-CSF mediated impairment of the liver to synthesize albumin, cholinesterase and cholesterol. *Am J Hematol.* **36**, 213–14.

Thompson JA, Lee DJ, Kidd P *et al.* (1989). Subcutaneous GM-CSF in patients with myelodysplastic syndrome: toxicity, pharmacokinetics, and hematological effects. *J Clin Oncol.* **7**, 629–37.

Vadhan-Raj S, Keating M, Lemaistre A *et al.* (1987). Effects of recombinant human GM-CSF in patients with myelodysplastic syndromes. *N Engl J Med.* **317**, 1545–52.

Vadhan-Raj S, Buescher S, Brozmeyer HE *et al.* (1988). Stimulation of myelopoiesis in patients with aplastic anemia by recombinant human GM-CSF. *N Engl J Med.* **319**, 1628.

Van Leeuwen BH, Martinson ME, Webb GC and Young IG (1989). Molecular organisation of the cytokine gene cluster, involving the human IL-3, IL-4, IL-5, and GM-CSF genes, on human chromosome 5. *Blood.* **73**, 1142.

49

Welte K, Zeidler C, Reiter A *et al.* (1990). Differential effects of GM-CSF and G-CSF in children with severe congenital neutropenia. *Blood.* **75**, 1056–63.

Williamson DJ, Begley CG, Vadas MA and Metcalf D (1988). The detection and initial characterization of colony-stimulating factors in synovial fluid. *Clin Exp Immunol.* **72**, 67.

Wong GG, Witek JS, Temple PA *et al.* (1985). Human GM–CSF: molecular cloning of the complementary DNA and purification of the natural and recombinant proteins. *Science.* **228**, 810.

4

GRANULOCYTE COLONY-STIMULATING FACTOR

F. TAKAKU

STRUCTURE, PRODUCTION AND FUNCTIONS

Granulocyte colony-stimulating factor (G-CSF) is a glycoprotein with a molecular weight of 19 kDa. This haematopoietic factor is one of the CSFs contained within the 'colony-stimulating activity' (CSA) that promotes myeloid colony growth in in vitro systems (first developed in the mid-1960s). Further studies have demonstrated that this CSA can be separated into at least four CSFs: multilineage (Multi-CSF, IL-3), granulocyte–macrophage (GM-CSF), macrophage (M-CSF), and granulocyte (G-CSF). The name of each CSF describes the type of colony growth which is promoted in the presence of that particular factor.

cDNA for G-CSF had been cloned independently by Souza *et al.* (1986) and Nagata *et al.* (1986) from two human tumour cell lines each producing human G-CSF in vitro. Production of recombinant human G-CSF (rhG-CSF) with the structure shown in Fig 4.1 was possible using *E. coli* or Chinese Hamster Ovary (CHO) cells (rhG-CSF produced by *E. coli* has no sugar moieties).

G-CSF is produced by macrophages, vascular endothelial cells, fibroblasts and certain malignant cells including human leukaemia myeloblasts. The production of G-CSF from macrophages had been shown to be stimulated by lipopolysaccharide (LPS) e.g. endotoxin.

Vascular endothelial cells and fibroblasts, on the other hand, produce G-CSF upon stimulation with interleukin-1 (IL-1) as well as tumour necrosis factor (TNF). Based on this mechanism of the production of G-CSF from various cells, it is speculated that in the event of a bacterial infection,

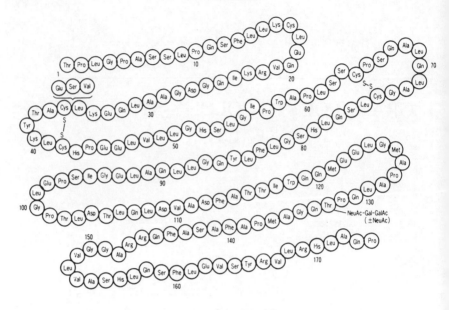

Fig. 4.1. Structure of G-CSF.

macrophages will produce G-CSF, IL-1 and TNF with the stimulation by bacterial endotoxin. The IL-1 and TNF thus produced will stimulate endothelial cells and fibroblasts to produce G-CSF. The accumulation of G-CSF in blood stimulates bone marrow cells to increase the production of neutrophils to protect the host against bacterial infections. It is evident from this chain of reactions, that G-CSF plays a key role in defence against bacterial infections.

Results of in vitro as well as in vivo studies with G-CSF have revealed, however, that G-CSF has other functions than the stimulation of the production of neutrophils in the bone marrow. As shown in Fig. 4.2, G-CSF had been shown to increase the production of neutrophils by increasing the numbers of multipotent, erythroid, granulocyte–macrophage and granulocyte precursors in bone marrow, probably in collaboration with other haematopoietic factors such as stem cell factor (SCF), interleukin-3 (IL-3), GM-CSF and others, although stimulation of granulocyte precursors is specific to G-CSF. G-CSF stimulates the release of mature neutrophils from bone marrow into peripheral blood. This function of G-CSF is demonstrated by the rapid increase of neutrophils in peripheral blood after the single intravenous administration of rhG-CSF to normal volunteers as shown in Fig. 4.3. The peripheral blood neutrophils start to increase as early as 4.5 h after an i.v administration of rhG-CSF and reach a maximum after 12.5 h. Functions of

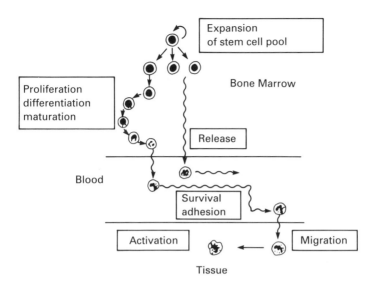

Fig. 4.2. In vivo activities of G-CSF.

mature neutrophils, such as migration, phagocytosis, production of superoxide anion and antibody dependent cytoxicity have been reported to be stimulated by in vitro as well as by in vivo experiments. From these observations, G-CSF is regarded as the key haematopoietic factor in the defence system operated by neutrophils. It stimulates the production, release and functions of neutrophils, as shown in Fig. 4.2.

G-CSF exerts its action through its specific receptor on the cell surface (the receptor has recently been cloned; Fukunaga *et al.*, 1990). Among various haematopoietic cells, only neutrophils and their precursors have the receptor for G-CSF. Therefore, the action of G-CSF is specific to cells of neutrophilic lineage. G-CSF does not stimulate the production of other types of granulocyte, monocytes, platelets and erythrocytes. Also, it does not stimulate the function of other types of granulocyte or monocytes.

CLINICAL APPLICATION OF G-CSF

As G-CSF had initially been identified as the factor to stimulate granulocyte colonies in vitro, it has long been questioned whether G-CSF has in vivo granulopoietic action as a granulopoietin. This question was answered as soon

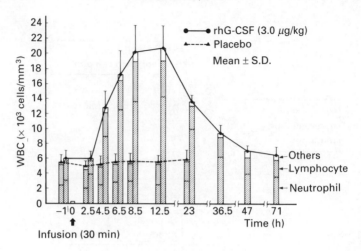

Fig. 4.3. Mean WBC count following intravenous infusion of rhG-CSF (3.0 mcg/kg) in normal healthy male volunteers ($n = 5$).

as enough rhG-CSF became available for in vivo studies. It is evident from the results shown in Fig. 4.3, that the administration of rhG-CSF can induce a marked increase in peripheral blood neutrophils. Repeated injections of rhG-CSF to patients with normal bone marrow function increased the peripheral blood neutrophil levels up to $50–60 \times 10^9/l$.

Two kinds of recombinant human G-CSF are available for clinical use, *E. coli* or CHO cell-derived agent. There are no significant differences in in vitro activities, clearance from plasma or in in vivo activities; they are equally efficacious clinically. Therefore, results of clinical studies obtained using both kinds of rhG-CSF will be presented in this essay without mentioning which rhG-CSF has been used.

Effect of rhG-CSF on neutropenia associated with cancer chemotherapy

From the results shown in Fig. 4.3, it is evident that rhG-CSF can increase neutrophils in peripheral blood. Therefore, neutropenias of various origins were considered as targets for the clinical trial of rhG-CSF. Chemotherapy-related neutropenia was selected as the first target for clinical trials. It is well documented that in most chemotherapy regimens, neutropenia is the dose-limiting factor. It is anticipated, therefore, that G-CSF will enable the administration of increasing doses of anticancer drugs and increase the cure rate of chemotherapy in various malignancies, thus improving quality of life and survival.

Non-Hodgkin's lymphoma

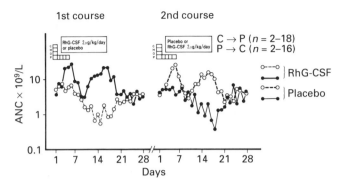

Fig. 4.4. Acceleration of ANC recovery by rhG-CSF administration in cancer patients after chemotherapy.

The types and doses of anticancer drugs are different for each patient. The degree of bone marrow suppression induced by anticancer drugs differs in each patient even after treatment with the same chemotherapy. Therefore, to study the effect of rhG-CSF on chemotherapy-related neutropenia, a cross-over study in which cancer patients received more than two courses of treatment with the same anticancer drugs, each followed by the administration of rhG-CSF or placebo (human albumin), was conducted to investigate the effect and the safety of rhG-CSF. Changes of peripheral blood neutrophil counts were compared between rhG-CSF and placebo periods. Figure 4.4 shows the results of a double-blind cross-over phase III trial in patients with non-Hodgkin's lymphoma, repeatedly treated with cyclophosphamide, Adriamycin, vincristine and prednisolone (CHOP) therapy. In this study, patients were allocated to one of two groups: either receiving rhG-CSF after the first CHOP treatment and placebo after the second treatment, or placebo after the first treatment and rhG-CSF after the second treatment.

Informed consent was obtained from patients prior to enrolment in the study. As shown in Fig. 4.4, the nadir of neutrophil counts after CHOP treatment was higher and recovery from neutropenia was earlier in the rhG-CSF-treated period than in the placebo-treated period, irrespective of whether the patients received rhG-CSF after the first or second course of chemotherapy. Days with fever over 38 °C were significantly fewer in the rhG-CSF-treated period as compared to placebo period. In treatment protocols containing methotrexate such as M-VAC (used in treatment of bladder carcinoma), Gabrilove *et al.* (1988) reported that the incidence and degree of stomatitis decreased significantly with the treatment with rhG-CSF. No difference was observed in the recovery of platelets, lymphocytes and reticulocytes between the rhG-CSF-treated period and placebo-treated period.

From the results described above, it is evident that by using rhG-CSF we can prevent the neutropenia following the administration of anticancer drugs and will be able to increase the doses of anticancer drugs to be given to patients irrespective of the kind of cancer. Higher response rates to anticancer treatment with increased dose of drugs have already been reported in combination with rhG-CSF treatment (Bronchud *et al.*, 1989). It is expected that the administration of rhG-CSF after treatment with anticancer drugs will become a standard therapy for cancer patients in the very near future. The administration of rhG-CSF for chemotherapy-related neutropenia has been approved by the FDA in the United States and CPMP in Europe.

In addition to the induction of neutrophilia, rhG-CSF has the remarkable characteristic of having almost no side-effects. Infrequent and transient bone pain can occur during administration of G-CSF, and this is easily treated with indomethacin. Other cytokines such as interferons, interleukins and GM-CSF seem to have rather more significant toxicities. Only erythropoietin is comparable to G-CSF in showing so few side-effects. This relative lack of toxicity may well encourage widespread use of G-CSF in cancer treatment.

The possibility of stimulating proliferation of solid tumour cells by G-CSF had been examined. However, results of a recent study suggest that the G-CSF receptor is very rarely present on the surface of tumour cells, thus making them relatively insensitive to the effects of the cytokine itself.

Effect of rhG-CSF on neutropenia after bone marrow transplantation

Allogeneic and autologous bone marrow transplantation is performed in many hospitals to treat patients with severe aplastic anaemia, leukaemia and congenital severe combined immunodeficiency or with various cancers responsive to chemotherapy and/or radiotherapy. The number of such patients receiving bone marrow transplantation has increased dramatically.

In both types of bone marrow transplantation, patients receive high-dose chemotherapy and/or immunosuppressive agents. Total body irradiation in addition to chemotherapy is often peformed. As the result of this conditioning, severe bone marrow failure occurs after transplantation, and it usually takes 3–4 weeks after transplantation before transplanted marrow stem cells engraft in the marrow of the recipient, and start to proliferate and

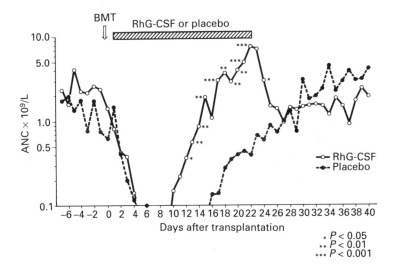

Fig. 4.5. Effects of rhG-CSF on neutrophil recovery after bone marrow transplantation.

differentiate to produce mature neutrophils. During these 3–4 weeks, the patient is highly susceptible to potentially life-threatening infections.

The clinical trial of rhG-CSF in patients receiving bone marrow transplantation has been conducted to investigate whether the administration of rhG-CSF can shorten this severely neutropenic period after bone marrow transplantation and reduce the incidence of infections occurring in this neutropenic period. The results of such a study, performed in a double-blind, placebo-controlled manner, are shown in Fig. 4.5 (Asano and Takaku, 1991). In this study, patients were given rhG-CSF (5 mcg/kg/day) or placebo intravenously every day for 21 consecutive days, starting one day after transplantation. As is clearly indicated in Fig. 4.5, patients receiving rhG-CSF showed an apparently earlier recovery from neutropenia after bone marrow transplantation than placebo-treated patients.

Percentages of patients with fever ($> 38\ °C$) after bone marrow transplantation were lower in rhG-CSF-treated groups than in placebo-treated groups as shown in Fig. 4.6. Numbers of days confined in isolation after bone marrow transplantation were also fewer in rhG-CSF than in placebo groups.

Whether we can reduce the total cost of bone marrow transplantation by using rhG-CSF is dependent upon the cost of rhG-CSF. In the United States rhG-CSF costs $108 (£64) per 300 mcg. If 5 mcg/kg are used for 21 days after transplantation, the total cost of rhG-CSF for one bone marrow

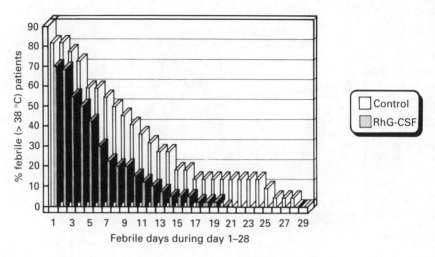

Fig. 4.6. Effects of G-CSF on fever after bone marrow transplantation.

transplantation will be over $2000 (£1176). If this is less than the cost of larger doses of antibiotics and a longer stay in transplant rooms, then rhG-CSF can reduce the cost for bone marrow transplantation. Tentative calculations have indicated a positive answer, it must not be forgotten that the most important benefit of rhG-CSF would be to increase the quality of life of the patient.

Concerns about increasing the incidence and severity of graft-versus-host disease (GVHD) associated with bone marrow transplantation by giving rhG-CSF have been voiced since the start of clinical trials. However, results of two clinical trials performed in Japan, each using non-glycosylated and glycosylated rhG-CSF, have shown that there was no difference in the incidence and severity of both acute and chronic GVHD between rhG-CSF-treated groups and placebo-treated groups.

rhG-CSF is also useful for autologous peripheral blood stem cell transplantation. It is well documented that multipotential stem cells are present in the circulation, and that they can be utilized in autologous peripheral blood stem cell transplantation to accelerate recovery. Several investigators have found that the numbers of such peripheral blood stem cells are increased with rhG-CSF in the setting of marrow recovery following chemotherapy. This acceleration is observed not only in granulocyte–macrophage precursors (CFU-GM) but in erythroid (BFU-E) and multilineage precursors (CFU-GEMM). The mechanism of this acceleration by rhG-CSF is not yet clear. Employing these properties of rhG-CSF, we propose a new protocol for cancer treatment, as shown in Fig. 4.7. In the conventional protocol shown in the upper part of Fig. 4.7, cancer

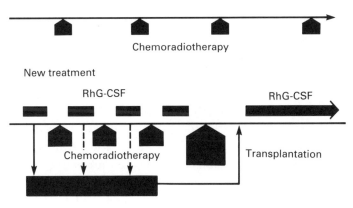

Fig. 4.7. A new chemotherapy protocol of cancer with rhG-CSF.

patients are treated repeatedly with conventional doses of anticancer drugs. Although present cancer chemotherapy strategies are designed to minimize drug resistance, patients will eventually become resistant to anticancer drugs unless they are cured by few courses of treatment. In a new treatment protocol shown in the lower part of Fig. 4.7, cancer patients are given rhG-CSF after each anticancer chemotherapy. With the administration of rhG-CSF, increasing doses of anticancer drugs can be administered because of the improvement in the nadir of neutrophil counts induced by rhG-CSF administration. The interval between chemotherapy administrations may also be shortened as a result of accelerated neutrophil recovery with rhG-CSF (see Fig. 4.4). It is proposed to collect peripheral blood stem cells and/or bone marrow cells at each chemotherapy cycle and store them. At the last chemotherapy, very large doses of anticancer drugs will be given to assure the disappearance of cancer cells, followed by the transfusion of stored stem cells. Patients will be further treated with larger doses of rhG-CSF to accelerate the recovery from severe neutropenia which is induced by the last large dose of chemotherapy. Other haematopoietic factors such as SCF, IL-3, GM-CSF and erythropoietin may also be employed in such a protocol, further accelerating the recovery of bone marrow failure and increasing the number of peripheral blood as well as bone marrow stem cells to be used for autologous transplantation.

This new protocol for cancer treatment using haematopoietic factor(s) and autologous stem cell transplantation is expected not only to improve the cure rate of cancer patients but also to increase the types of cancer that can be effectively treated with chemotherapy.

Effect of rhG-CSF on other neutropenias

rhG-CSF can increase the number of peripheral blood neutrophils in about 60% of the patients with aplastic anaemia. This increase was confined to neutrophils and limited only to the period of rhG-CSF administration. Soon after the termination of the administration of rhG-CSF, the increased neutrophil counts returned to pretreatment levels. Preliminary results of a multi-institutional clinical trial performed in Japan showed that only aplastic anaemia patients with neutrophil counts $> 0.1 \times 10^9$/l can effectively respond to rhG-CSF administration. Although the effect of rhG-CSF is transient and usually limited to patients with some bone marrow reserve, rhG-CSF is worth a trial in patients with aplastic anaemia with infections. Preliminary results of clinical trials have indicated the effectiveness of rhG-CSF in such patients.

Another disorder in which the clinical efficacy of rhG-CSF has been studied is the myelodysplastic syndrome (MDS). In this disorder, it is well documented that neutropenia often develops in addition to anaemia and thrombocytopenia, and that neutrophil function is often defective. Infection and transformation to acute myelogenous leukaemia are the two main causes of death in MDS patients. Results of a multi-institutional clinical trial revealed that almost all patients with MDS, except those developing acute leukaemia, respond to rhG-CSF with a significant increase of peripheral blood neutrophil counts (Negrin *et al.*, 1990). Decreased neutrophil alkaline phosphatase (NAP) activity, which is often observed in patients with MDS, recovered to a normal level by incubating the patients' neutrophils in vitro with rhG-CSF or after an in vivo administration of rhG-CSF to patients for 7–14 days. It is expected, therefore, that rhG-CSF can prevent or treat the infections that often occur in patients with MDS through an increase in neutrophil counts and through the recovery of decreased neutrophil functions. However, the use of rhG-CSF in patients with MDS classified as refractory anaemia with excess of blasts (RAEB) or RAEB in transformation (RAEB-t) requires great care, as these patients have higher percentages of marrow myeloblasts. Such patients may be prone to develop acute myelogenous leukaemia as myeloblasts possess the receptor for G-CSF and GM-CSF, and therefore G-CSF could potentially promote myeloblast growth.

rhG-CSF has been shown to be effective in various types of congenital and acquired neutropenia. In congenital neutropenia accompanied by defective neutrophil functions, such as type Ib glycogen storage disease, administration of rhG-CSF resulted in the recovery of numbers, as well as of various neutrophil functions. Children with cyclic neutropenia responded to rhG-CSF administration with a higher nadir and peak neutrophil levels than pretreatment values. Although cycling of blood cell counts continued, the neutrophil nadir was less marked after the start of rhG-CSF administration, and the condition of patients was markedly improved during rhG-CSF (Hammond *et al.*, 1989).

Most of the congenital or idiopathic neutropenias occur in children and have a chronic course. Therefore, patients may need life-long G-CSF administration. As these patients do not usually have thrombocytopenia, subcutaneous administration of rhG-CSF is possible and, using this method of administration, the amount of rhG-CSF necessary to maintain a normal peripheral blood neutrophil count can be reduced to less than one-half of that necessary for intravenous administration.

Use of rhG-CSF in leukaemia treatment

As in the case of treatment of solid tumours by anticancer drugs, rhG-CSF administration can accelerate neutrophil recovery after antileukaemia chemotherapy (Ohno *et al.*, 1990). There was no evidence that the administration of rhG-CSF accelerated regrowth of leukaemia cells or relapse in these patients.

Leukaemic myeloblasts possess the G-CSF receptor and proliferate in response to G-CSF in vitro. There is evidence that human leukaemic myeloblasts also respond to G-CSF in vivo. Utilizing these properties, we conducted a clinical trial to treat refractory or relapsed acute myelogenous leukaemia patients with the combination of rhG-CSF and antileukaemic drugs. It was expected that refractory leukaemic cells, which are often dormant, would be stimulated to proliferate by G-CSF and become sensitive to cycle-specific antileukacmic drugs such as cytosine arabinoside, as shown in Fig. 4.8. Results of preliminary clinical studies have shown that some patients with acute myelogenous leukaemia who have become resistant to antileukaemia drugs can achieve complete responses to the combination of G-CSF and chemotherapy. Although the duration of complete remission of such patients is usually short, such combinations may be worth trying in resistant cases. Other haemopoietic factors, such as IL-3, GM-CSF or combinations of these factors with G-CSF, have been reported to be much more effective in stimulating the dormant leukaemic myeloblasts to go into cell cycle. If the combination of these haematopoietic factors does not induce severe side-effects, such combinations may be coupled with antileukaemia drugs to further improve cell responsiveness.

A trial to treat refractory acute myelogenous leukaemia patients with the combination of rhG-CSF and antileukaemia drugs with or without the addition of total body irradiation as conditioning for bone marrow

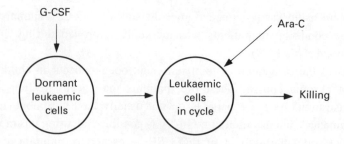

Fig. 4.8. Combination of G-CSF and antileukaemia agents for the treatment of refractory myelogenous leukaemia.

transplantation has also been conducted. The rationale for treatment with a combination of rhG-CSF and antileukaemia drugs in refractory myelogenous leukaemia is the same as that described above. However, in this trial a higher dose of drugs was used and, in some patients, total irradiation was performed. Following such supralethal therapies, bone marrow transplantation followed by administration of rhG-CSF was necessary as rescue. Results indicated that the prognosis of the refractory myelogenous leukaemia cases treated with G-CSF was better than that of historical controls who were conditioned for transplantation without G-CSF.

Use of rhG-CSF for treatment of intractable infections

G-CSF stimulates neutrophil functions. This property has been employed in the treatment of intractable infections such as AIDS or infections occurring in elderly people.

The neutropenia of AIDS improves following G-CSF administration, and this is often associated with improvement in fever. There are case reports on the effectiveness of rhG-CSF on the various intractable infections that occur in the compromised host. This effect is attributed to the activity of G-CSF to stimulate the production and functions of neutrophils. However, well-designed clinical studies are needed to show the usefulness of rhG-CSF in intractable infections.

CONCLUSION

rhG-CSF is one of the most exciting drugs to have been developed during the past decade. Its development became possible only through the progress in biotechnological techniques and, in this regard, clinicians and patients owe a great deal to scientists in the field of molecular biology.

As described, rhG-CSF is a unique cytokine, the action of which is limited mostly to the cells of the neutrophilic series. It has several clinical uses and is relatively non-toxic. The accumulation of clinical experience with rhG-CSF may further extend the range of utility of this agent.

REFERENCES

Asano S and Takaku F (1991). Beneficial effect of recombinant human glycosylated granulocyte colony-stimulating factor in marrow-transplanted patients: results of multicentre phase II-III studies. *Transplantation Proceed.* **23**, 1701–3.

Bronchud MH, Howell A, Crowther D *et al.* (1989). The use of granulocyte colony-stimulating factor to increase the intensity of treatment with Doxorubicin in patients with advanced breast and ovarian cancer. *Brit J Cancer.* **60**, 121–5.

Fukunaga R, Ishizaka-Ikeda E and Nagata S (1990). Purification and characterisation of the receptor for murine granulocyte colony-stimulating factor. *J Biol Chem.* **265**, 1408–15.

Gabrilove JL, Jakubowski A, Scher H *et al.* (1988). Effect of granulocyte colony stimulating factor on neutropenia and associated morbidity due to chemotherapy for transitional-cell carcinoma of the urothelium. *New Engl J Med.* **318**, 1414–22.

Hammond WP, Price TH, Souza LM *et al.* (1989). Treatment of cyclic neutropenia with granylocyte colony-stimulating factor. *New Engl J Med.* **320**, 1306–11.

Nagata S, Tsuchiya M, Asano S *et al.* (1986). Molecular cloning and expression of cDNA for human granulocyte colony-stimulating factor. *Nature.* **319**, 415–8.

Negrin SR, Haeuber DH, Nagler A *et al.* (1990). Maintenance treatment of patients with myelodysplastic syndromes using recombinant hG-CSF. *Blood.* **75**, 36–43.

Ohno R, Tomonaga M, Kobayashi T *et al.* (1990). Effect of granulocyte colony-stimulating factor after intensive induction therapy in relapsed or refractory acute leukaemia. *New Engl J Med.* **323**, 871–7.

Souza LM, Boone TC, Gabrilove JL *et al.* (1986). Recombinant human granulocyte colony-stimulating factor: Effects on normal and leukaemic myeloid cells. *Science.* **232**, 61–5.

5

INTERLEUKIN-1

G. C. BAGBY, Jr

INTRODUCTION

The availability of the genes encoding haematopoietic growth factors and their receptors has empowered us to test exactly how a given change in the environment incites expression of the proper human genes at precisely the appropriate time. Results of therapeutic trials in which such factors have been administered to experimental animals (and also to humans) demonstrate responses that were predicted in advance by investigators with experience using in vitro techniques. Thus, these in vivo observations have validated in vitro assays as verifiable windows through which naturally occurring in vivo events can be observed.

Unfortunately, what we see through these windows is increasingly complex. Models of the inflammatory response are orders of magnitude more perplexing than certain other models in haematopoiesis. Regulation of erythropoiesis, for example, can be comprehended as a relatively tight package. Hypoxia results in an increase in erythropoietin synthesis (Stohlman et al., 1954; Goldberg et al., 1988) and this glycoprotein hormone induces lineage-specific proliferation and differentiation of cells of the erythroid lineage (Semenza et al., 1989). The response to microbial stressors, however, is tremendously complicated, partly because each organ system must have a capacity to serve a sentinel role, and partly because so many arms of the immune and haematopoietic systems must be recruited to participate in the response.

So that they will not be startled by the spectrum of biological responses and toxicities induced in their patients by the administration of interleukins and haematopoietic growth factors, all physicians should possess a working knowledge of the basic types of complexities associated with these factors.

Table 5.1. *Biological complexities of the cytokine network*

Growth factors and interleukins exhibit heterogeneous biological activities.

Proteins that induce proliferation of specific hematopoietic progenitor cells often activate the functional capacity of the differentiated daughter cells of the same lineage.

Haematopoietic growth factors and interleukins can act directly on effector cells of inflammation or indirectly on them through effects on intermediary cells.

Specific growth factors and interleukins commonly act synergistically with others.

The network of growth factors and interleukins involved in the inflammatory response is organized hierarchically.

Autoamplification loops are common in the cytokine network.

The majority are summarized in Table 5.1. Interleukin-1 (IL-1) serves as a perfect paradigm of the 'rules' outlined in Table 5.1

STRUCTURE AND BIOLOGICAL ACTIVITY OF IL-1

IL-1, formerly known as endogenous pyrogen and lymphocyte-activating factor, exists in two molecular forms (IL-1α and IL-1β) encoded by two genes on chromosome 2 (Webb *et al.*, 1986; Lafage *et al.*, 1989). Each of these is a 31 kDa precursor molecule which is cleaved to a 17 kDa peptide. IL-1 can be produced by almost all cells. Expression of the genes is induced by endotoxin, IL-1, granulocyte–macrophage colony-stimulating factor (GM-CSF), tumour necrosis factor (TNF) and IL-2. The IL-1 receptor, which binds both forms of IL-1 (Chin *et al.*, 1988; Dinarello *et al.*, 1989a), is a 60–70 kDa protein of the immunoglobulin superfamily (Sims *et al.*, 1988) encoded by a gene also found on chromosome 2 (Copeland *et al.*, 1991). The bioactivity of IL-1 is broad and there is good evidence that it regulates most processes involved in inflammation (Table 5.2).

The broad activity of IL-1 derives, in large part, from its ability to induce the expression of other interleukin and CSF genes which themselves function as subordinate effector molecules in the inflammatory process. For example, IL-1 has no capacity to directly induce proliferation of granulocyte progenitor cells in vitro, but, when administered in vivo, universally induces neutrophilic leucocytosis which results from the induction of G-CSF and GM-CSF expression by other cells, including fibroblasts (Lee *et al.*, 1987; Fibbe *et al.*,

Table 5.2. *The structure and function of interleukin-1*

Synonym: endogenous pyrogen, LAF, LAM, others
Chromosomal location: 2q
Gene product: 31 kDa precursor, 17 kDa cleavage product
Produced by: most cells
Induced by: endotoxin, IL-1, GM-CSF, TNFα, IL-2
Receptor: 60-70 kDa, immunoglobulin superfamily
Representative biological functions:

　A. Induces expression of GM-CSF, G-CSF, IL-6 and IL-1 in fibroblasts,
　　　endothelial cells, keratinocytes and thymic epithelial cells (Bagby, 1989)
　B. Induces proliferation of pre-activated T cells (Lichtman *et al.*, 1988)
　C. Induces acute-phase protein synthesis (Dinarello, 1988; Mortensen, 1988)
　D. Induces fever and sleep in vivo (Dinarello and Savage, 1989)
　E. Stimulates release of ACTH (Lumpkin, 1987; Sapolsky *et al.*, 1987)
　F. Promotes transendothelial passage of neutrophils (Moser *et al.*, 1989)
　G. Synergizes with IL-3 in stimulating proliferation in primitive haematopoietic
　　　progenitor cells in vitro (Bartelmez *et al.*, 1989)
　H. Stimulates prostaglandin E production in fibroblasts, monocytes and
　　　neutrophils (Zucali *et al.*, 1986; Elias *et al.*, 1987; Conti *et al.*, 1988)
　I. Modulates EGF receptor expression (Bird and Saklatvala, 1989)

1988; Seelentag *et al.*, 1989), endothelial cells (Segal and Bagby, 1988; Segal *et al.*, 1988; Zsebo *et al.*, 1988), thymic epithelial cells (Ridgway *et al.*, 1988) and T lymphocytes (Herrmann *et al.*, 1988). The impact of IL-1 on other components of the inflammatory response is similarly controlled; that is, indirectly through the actions of IL-6, IL-8, G-CSF, endothelial–leucocyte adhesion molecule-1 (ELAM-1) and intercellular adhesion molecule-1 (ICAM-1) (Bagby and Segal, 1991). The central role of IL-1 in regulation of the inflammatory response serves as an obvious example of the hierarchy rule (Table 5.1) (Bagby, 1989).

　Certain haematopoietic growth factors and interleukins can act both directly and indirectly. That is, some of the peptides with haematopoietic activity directly stimulate growth and/or proliferation of one cell type but, in other cells, the same proteins induce expression of other growth-factor genes and, thus, act indirectly. IL-2 and GM-CSF, for example, directly induce proliferative responses in lymphocytes and myeloid progenitors (CFU-GM) respectively, but also induce expression of IL-1 by auxiliary cells (Numerof *et al.*, 1988; Sisson and Dinarello, 1988). To make matters worse, IL-1 is capable of enhancing expression of itself (Warner *et al.*, 1987; Mauviel *et al.*, 1988) and another hierarchically important indirect-acting acute-phase response protein, TNFα, can also induce IL-1 gene expression (Nawroth *et al.*, 1986; Le *et al.*, 1987). Therefore, IL-1 itself induces IL-1 gene expression and the gene is also induced by proteins that IL-1 itself induces (Lindemann *et al.*, 1988; Bagby, 1989). This latter phenomenon has been validated in humans receiving recombinant GM-CSF who were found to have high levels of TNFα, IL-1 and IL-6 mRNA in their alveolar macrophages. Thus, such signal amplification mechanisms can be autocrine, paracrine, or both.

These considerations have enormous importance to our understanding of the expected biological effects of IL-1 therapy and also provide clues for side-effects, some of which might be expected to worsen the underlying disease under study. Those of us involved in clinical study-design are obliged to ensure that all of the proteins induced by the recombinant therapeutic factor used are quantified and their potential adverse effects tested, when possible, in advance of therapy.

EXPERIMENTAL THERAPY WITH IL-1

Because of its capacity to influence immunological reactivity, the inflammatory response and haematopoiesis, a number of preclinical trials of IL-1 have been carried out. Three experimental situations are highlighted: radiation injury, cancer therapy and systemic infections.

Radiation injury

In 1987, Schwartz *et al.* reported that mice treated with recombinant IL-1α either before or after sublethal or lethal radiation demonstrated in vitro signs of early haematopoietic recovery. Specifically, after 8 to 12 days postradiation, there was a noticeable increase in the number of committed progenitor cells and CFU-S (a multipotential progenitor cell) in the treated animals. In addition, they noted that the proliferative activity (fraction in S-phase of the cell cycle) of committed granulocyte progenitor cells increased after IL-1 administration. While at first such effects were ascribed to the capacity of IL-1 to enhance synthesis of haematopoietic growth factors by marrow stromal cells, later studies have suggested that this explanation may not suffice to explain the phenomenon in its entirety. That is, Neta (1990) have shown that postradiation administration of G-CSF or GM-CSF does not mimic the radioprotective effect of IL-1. This result could be attributed to the design of the studies, which did not include all IL-1-inducible haematopoietic growth factors (e.g. adhesion molecules or IL-6), or to the capacity for IL-1 to induce expression or activation of scavenger proteins that function to limit radiation-induced oxidative injury (White and Ghezzi, 1989; Neta, 1990). Additional evidence in support of the use of IL-1 in modulating radiation injury derives from the recent studies of Wu and Miyamoto (1990), documenting that IL-1 is capable of protecting gut epithelium from radiation-induced injury.

It is most remarkable that postradiation therapy with IL-1 is capable of abrogating injury, a finding that has a good amount of clinical relevance for the management of radiation injury in humans. Unresolved issues of importance include the potential for IL-1 to induce radioresistance in the tumour for which radiation is being prescribed. Although one encouraging preliminary report has found that such tumour radioresistance is not induced by IL-1 (Dorie *et al.*, 1989), clearly further studies are warranted on this point.

Cancer therapy

Apart from its effect on radiation injury, two additional attributes of IL-1 have been investigated in the setting of cancer; its capacity to hasten recovery from antitumour chemotherapy, and its capacity to enhance antitumour immunity.

Recovery from myelosuppression IL-1 hastens recovery of the marrow in mice treated with 5-fluorouracil (5-FU) (Moore and Warren, 1987), cyclophosphamide (Stork *et al.*, 1989) and Adriamycin (Eppstein *et al.*, 1989). In addition, normal human haematopoietic progenitor cells are protected from injury by 4-hydroperoxy-cyclophosphamide (4-HC) (Moreb *et al.*, 1989) yet leukaemic cells seem not to be protected by IL-1 (Moreb *et al.*, 1989), an observation that is of particular interest to bone marrow transplanters using 4-HC in marrow purging for autologous marrow transplantation.

Thus, it seems clear that IL-1 is capable of protecting haematopoietic cells exposed to myelosuppressive agents from injury and death. These observations have caused a great deal of enthusiasm in the clinical oncology community for the design of new trials of anticancer therapy which include doses of myelosuppressive drugs previously considered to be lethal. This enthusiasm must be tempered by the recognition that increasing the dose-intensity of chemotherapeutic agents may have no effect on disease-free or overall survival in most malignancies. Therefore, for such studies to be clinically relevant to the design of new anticancer therapies, they must be validated in tumour-bearing animals in which the importance of dose-intensity can be readily tested.

Promising preliminary studies in animals bearing syngeneic tumours indicate that IL-1 seems to enhance antitumour drug effects in mice receiving mitomycin C, doxorubicin, cisplatinum, cyclophosphamide, or 5-FU (Nakamura et al., 1991). In addition, this same group demonstrated that at optimal doses of IL-1 (0.3–3.0 µg/mouse) certain mice bearing syngeneic colorectal carcinomas and treated with carboplatin or thiotepa were cured. Whether the effects on tumour therapy in this study derived from the well described haematopoietic effects of IL-1, from the capacity of IL-1 to prevent fatal infections in anticancer drug-treated mice (Morikage et al., 1990), or from its capacity to serve as a co-factor for tumour toxicity, is unknown at this time. Nonetheless, the potential value of IL-1 in the chemotherapeutic management of cancer patients may prove to be as great as it might prove to be in patients receiving radiation therapy.

Direct antitumour effects of IL-1 Recent evidence published by Belardelli et al. (1989) and Johnson et al. (1990) demonstrated that IL-1 can cause regression of Friend virus-induced erythroleukaemia. Johnson et al. (1990) report that IL-1 suppressed growth of leukaemic erythroid colony forming cells and induced regression of disease temporarily. Belardelli et al. (1989) found that subcutaneous injections of mice with IL-1 increased survival time and inhibited leukaemic growth in liver and spleen. In addition, combination therapy with IL-1 and IL-2 synergistically reduced tumour cell growth and, indeed, resulted in 60% survival of mice injected with highly aggressive Friend cells. A similar synergistic effect of IL-1 and IL-2 has been seen in mice implanted with Lewis lung carcinoma and the adenocarcinoma cell line 755 (Iigo et al., 1990). In the Belardelli study, the effect of IL-1 plus IL-2 was seen neither in leukaemic animals injected with antibodies to Thy 1.2 antigen nor in nude mice transplanted with the same tumour cells. Therefore, in this model, the cytostatic effect of this combination was clearly mediated, at least in part, by antitumour T lymphocytes. Other investigators have reported that IL-1 does have an effect on human lymphoma cells transplanted in nude mice (Miyamoto and Wu, 1990) so the role of T lymphocytes in the IL-1 response may differ between tumours and may depend upon the inclusion of IL-2 therapy with IL-1 therapy. The observations in the Friend system are particularly encouraging. Taking into account the strong evidence supporting the notion of the graft-versus-leukaemia effect (Anasetti et al., 1990; Bacigalupo et al., 1991) it is appealing to speculate that IL-1/IL-2 therapy of patients with acute non-lymphocytic leukaemia might be a rational approach to the induction of a similar T-cell-mediated antitumour effect in patients who are not transplant candidates.

Infectious diseases

Because of the master-switch role played by IL-1 in regulating the inflammatory response, a number of investigators have tested its efficacy in prevention and treatment of fungal, viral and bacterial infections. These studies have focused, in particular, upon infectious processes that are usually difficult to eradicate, in some cases because the infection involves animals whose inflammatory response is blunted (e.g. neutropenic animals (Van't Wout *et al.*, 1988; Nakamura *et al.*, 1989; Morikage *et al.*, 1990) or animals with thermal injury (Silver *et al.*, 1990)), and in others because the organism itself is particularly virulent or difficult to eradicate with antibiotics alone (van der Meer *et al.*, 1989a; Morikage *et al.*, 1990; Zhan *et al.*, 1991).

Van't Wout *et al.* (1988) demonstrated that pretreatment of neutropenic mice with recombinant IL-1 prevented lethal infection with *Candida albicans*. Similar observations were made when *Pseudomonas* was used as the infecting organism (van der Meer *et al.*, 1989b). Nakamura *et al.* (1989) found that IL-1 seemed to act synergistically with antibiotics (ceftazidime, moxalactam, gentamicin, enoxacin, and amphotericin B) in hastening antimicrobial responses in both neutropenic mice infected with *Pseudomonas* and non-neutropenic mice infected with a variety of species (*Pseudomonas aeruginosa, Klebsiella pneumoniae* and *Candida albicans*). Zhan *et al.* (1991) found that IL-1 treatment of mice prior to or soon after infection by *Brucella abortus* reduced growth of bacteria in the reticuloendothelial system, but that a similar effect was not seen in chronically infected animals. Because IL-1 enhanced the entry and/or production of neutrophils and monocytes in the spleen of acutely infected mice but did not effect this change in chronically infected mice, it is reasonable to propose that the production and activation of phagocytes accounted for this difference. Whether the failure of IL-1 to effect a reduction in the load of bacteria reflected a high endogenous IL-1 production rate in the chronically infected animals, or the production of proteins that inhibit the biological activity of IL-1 (Dinarello, 1991) has not been examined. IL-1, fully competent on its own, is also capable of enhancing TNFα-induced antibacterial resistance (Roll *et al.*, 1990) and protects mice against lethal cerebral malaria (Dinarello *et al.*, 1989b; Curfs *et al.*, 1990).

TOXICITY OF IL-1

Most clinical trials involving recombinant proteins address the problems of acute toxicities. In the case of IL-1 therapy, most of these are completely predictable and based upon the well known biological activities of this factor (Table 5.2). Because IL-1 has so many heterogeneous effects (induced by the myriad genes regulated by IL-1), the toxicities are diverse and include fever, myalgia, headache, anorexia, fatigue, leucocytosis, hypotension, shock (Okusawa *et al.*, 1988; Wakabayashi *et al.*, 1991) and weight loss.

Fewer trials in cancer patients address an equally important question, one that takes much more time to answer; will IL-1 therapy worsen the patient's neoplastic disease and hasten their ultimate demise? Is this a picky, irrelevant theoretical question? I argue that it is not. A number of investigative groups, including our own, have documented that certain recombinant haematopoietic growth factors stimulate the growth of cancer cells in vitro (Berdel *et al.*, 1989; Salmon and Liu, 1989). Clearly, if agents such as IL-1 permit more aggressive chemotherapy, one can only expect, at least in the short-term, some sort of tumour regression for sensitive tumours. Nonetheless, IL-1 induces expression of GM-CSF, G-CSF and IL-6, each of which can serve as an inducer of tumour cell growth. Thus, the increase in fractional tumour cell kill may be offset, in some cases, by an equivalent increase in the rate of tumour cell regrowth. This would be of particular concern in tumours known to proliferate reliably under the influence of IL-1-induced factors. Take myeloma as a case in point. Myeloma cells not only proliferate in response to IL-6, but commonly produce IL-6, which serves as an autocrine growth factor for these cells (Kawano *et al.*, 1989; Suematsu *et al.*, 1990). Treatment of myeloma patients with high dose drug therapy and/or radiation combined with IL-1 might permit a greater initial cell kill, but also permit more rapid regrowth. This might be clearly observed in clinical studies designed to examine this potential problem, but no studies to date have been published with this in mind. Not only do most clinical studies ask shorter-term questions, but, shockingly, some are even designed with so-called 'cross-over' strategies (by which patients in the control group who suffer myelosuppressive toxicity can subsequently receive the recombinant haematopoietic growth factor). Naturally, if all studies are designed in this way, we will never really know whether all this therapeutic intensity permitted by recombinant haematopoietic growth factors and interleukins is really warranted at all. The reader should bear in mind that IL-1-inducible proteins can stimulate the growth of a variety of neoplastic cells (Cozzolino *et al.*, 1989; Kawano *et al.*, 1989; Oster *et al.*, 1989; Bradbury *et al.*, 1990; Brandt *et al.*, 1990). For these reasons, I suggest that all therapeutic trials involving one or more haematopoietic growth factors or interleukins in cancer or leukaemia patients follow a few basic rules: (1) do not use a cross-over design, (2) test the responsiveness of the neoplastic cells obtained at the time of diagnosis in an in vitro proliferation assay (e.g. tumour cell colony growth, fluorescence cell cycle analysis, or Thd incorporation) prior to therapy, (cells should be cultured in the presence and absence of autologous peripheral blood mononuclear leukocytes to test for paracrine effects of the factor), (3) carry out long-term follow up with a study population large enough to permit meaningful analysis of overall benefits as measured by overall and disease-free survival.

REFERENCES

Anasetti C, Beatty PG, Storb R et al. (1990). Effect of HLA incompatibility on graft-versus-host disease, relapse, and survival after marrow transplantation for patients with leukemia or lymphoma. Hum Immunol. 29, 79–91.

Bacigalupo A, Van Lint MT, Occhini D et al. (1991). Increased risk of leukemia relapse with high-dose cyclosporine A after allogeneic marrow transplantation for acute leukemia. Blood. 77, 1423–8.

Bagby GC (1989). Interleukin 1 and hematopoiesis. Blood Rev. 3, 152–61.

Bagby GC, Dinarello CA, Wallace P et al. (1986). Interleukin-1 stimulates granulocyte macrophage colony stimulating activity release by vascular endothelial cells. J Clin Invest. 78, 1316–23.

Bagby GC and Segal GM (1991). Growth factors and the control of hematopoiesis. In: Hematology. Basic principles and practice, ed. Hoffman R, Benz EJ, Shattil SJ, Furie B and Cohen HJ, 97–121. New York: Churchill Livingstone Inc.

Bartelmez SH, Bradley TR, Bertoncello I et al. (1989). Interleukin 1 plus interleukin 3 plus colony-stimulating factor 1 are essential for clonal proliferation of primitive myeloid bone marrow cells. Exp Hematol. 17, 240–5.

Belardelli F, Ciolli V, Testa U et al. (1989). Anti-tumor effects of interleukin-2 and interleukin-1 in mice transplanted with different syngeneic tumors. Int J Cancer. 44, 1108–16.

Berdel WE, Danhauser-Riedl S, Steinhauser G and Winton EF (1989). Various human hematopoietic growth factors (interleukin- 3, GM-CSF, G-CSF) stimulate clonal growth of nonhematopoietic tumor cells. Blood. 73, 80–3.

Berkenbosch F, van Oers J, del Rey A et al. (1987). Corticotropin-releasing factor-producing neurons in the rat activated by interleukin-1. Science. 238, 524–6.

Bird TA and Saklatvala J (1989). IL-1 and TNF transmodulate epidermal growth factor receptors by a protein kinase C-independent mechanism. J Immunol. 142, 126–33.

Bradbury D, Rogers S, Kozlowski R et al. (1990). Interleukin-1 is one factor which regulates autocrine production of GM-CSF by the blast cells of acute myeloblastic leukaemia. Br J Haematol. 76, 488–93.

Brandt SJ, Bodine DM, Dunbar CE and Nienhuis AW (1990). Dysregulated interleukin-6 expression produces a syndrome resembling Castleman's disease in mice. J Clin Invest. 86, 592–9.

Chin J, Rupp E, Cameron PM *et al.* (1988). Identification of a high-affinity receptor for interleukin-1 alpha and interleukin-1 beta on cultured human rheumatoid synovial cells. *J Clin Invest.* **82**, 420–6.

Conti P, Reale M, Fiore S *et al.* (1988). Recombinant interleukin-1 and tumor necrosis factor acting in synergy to release thromboxane, 6-KETO-PGF1α and PGE2 by human neutrophils. *Scand J Rheumatol.* **17 (Suppl. 75)**, 318–24.

Copeland NG, Silan CM, Kingsley DM *et al.* (1991). Chromosomal location of murine and human IL-1 receptor genes. *Genomics.* **9**, 44–50.

Cozzolino F, Rubartelli A, Aldinucci D *et al.* (1989). Interleukin-1 as an autocrine growth factor for acute myeloid leukemia cells. *Proc Natl Acad Sci USA.* **86**, 2369–73.

Curfs JHAJ, van der Meer JWM, Sauerwein RW and Eling WMC (1990). Low dosages of interleukin-1 protect mice against lethal cerebral malaria. *J Exp Med.* **172**, 1287–91.

Dinarello CA (1988). Biology of interleukin-1. *FASEB J.* **2**, 108–15.

Dinarello CA (1991). Interleukin-1 and interleukin-1 antagonism. *Blood* 77, 1627–52.

Dinarello CA and Savage N (1989). Interleukin-1 and its receptor. *CRC Crit Rev Immunol.* **9**, 1–20.

Dinarello CA, Clark BD, Puren AJ, Savage N and Rosoff PM (1989a). The interleukin-1 receptor. *Immunol Today.* **10**, 49–51.

Dinarello CA, Okusawa S and Gelfand JA (1989b). Interleukin-1 induces a shock-like state in rabbits: synergism with tumor necrosis factor and the effect of cyclooxygenase inhibition. *Prog Clin Biol Res.* **286**, 243–63.

Dorie MJ, Allison AC, Zaghloul MS and Kallman RF (1989). Interleukin-1 protects against the lethal effects of irradiation of mice but has no effect on tumors in the same animals. *Proc Soc Exp Biol Med.* **191**, 23–9.

Elias JA, Gustilo K, Baeder W and Freundlich B (1987). Synergistic stimulation of fibroblast prostaglandin production by recombinant interleukin-1 and tumor necrosis factor. *J Immunol.* **138**, 3812–16.

Eppstein DA, Kurahara CG, Bruno, NA and Terrell TG (1989). Prevention of doxorubicin-induced hematotoxicity in mice by interleukin 1. *Cancer Res.* **49**, 3955–60.

Fibbe WE, Van Damme J and Billiau A (1988). Human fibroblasts produce granulocyte-CSF, macrophage-CSF, and granulocyte-macrophage-CSF following stimulation by interleukin-1 and poly(rI).poly(rC). *Blood.* **72**, 860–6.

Goldberg MA, Dunning SP and Bunn HF (1988). Regulation of the erythropoietin gene: Evidence that the oxygen sensor is a heme protein. *Science.* **242**, 1412–15.

Herrmann F, Oster W, Meuer SC *et al.* (1988). Interleukin-1 stimulates T lymphocytes to produce granulocyte-monocyte colony-stimulating factor. *J Clin Invest.* **81**, 1415–18.

Iigo M, Nishikata K and Hoshi A (1990). Effect of recombinant interleukin-1 alpha, recombinant interleukin-2, recombinant interferon-beta, and recombinant tumor necrosis factor on subcutaneously implanted adenocarcinoma 755 and Lewis lung carcinoma. *J Biol Response Mod.* **9**, 426–30.

Johnson CS, Chang MJ, Thurlow SM *et al.* (1990). Immunotherapeutic approaches to leukemia: the use of the Friend virus-induced erythroleukemia model system. *Cancer Res.* **50**, 5682S–86S.

Kawano M, Tanaka H, Ishikawa H *et al.* (1989). Interleukin-1 accelerates autocrine growth of myeloma cells through interleukin-6 in human myeloma. *Blood.* **73**, 2145–48.

Lafage M, Maroc N, Dubreuil P *et al.* (1989). The human interleukin-1a gene is located on the long arm of chromosome 2 at band q13. *Blood.* **73**, 104–7.

Larrick JW (1989). Native interleukin-1 inhibitors. *Immunol Today.* **10**, 61–6.

Le JM, Weinstein D, Gubler U and Vilcek J (1987). Induction of membrane-associated interleukin 1 by tumor necrosis factor in human fibroblasts. *J.Immunol.* **138**, 2137–42.

Lee M, Segal, GM, and Bagby GC (1987). Interleukin-1 induces human bone marrow-derived fibroblasts to produce multilineage hematopoietic growth factors. *Exp Hematol.* **15**, 983–8.

Lichtman AH, Chin J, Schmidt JA and Abbas AK (1988). Role of interleukin-1 in the activation of T lymphocytes. *Proc Natl Acad Sci USA.* **85**, 9699–9703.

Lindemann A, Riedel D, Oster W *et al.* (1988). Granulocyte/macrophage colony-stimulating factor induces interleukin 1 production by human polymorphonuclear neutrophils. *J Immunol.* **140**, 837–9.

Lumpkin MD (1987). The regulation of ACTH secretion by IL-1. *Science.* **238**, 452–4.

Mauviel A, Temime N, Charron D *et al.* (1988). Interleukin-1 a and induce interleukin-1 gene expression in human dermal fibroblasts. *Biochem Biophys Res Commun.* **156**, 1209–14.

Miyamoto T and Wu SG (1990). Antitumor activity of recombinant human interleukin-1 against heterotransplanted human non-Hodgkin lymphomas in nude mice. *Jpn J Cancer Res.* **81**, 1175–83.

Moore MAS and Warren DJ (1987). Synergy of interleukin 1 and granulocyte colony-stimulating factor: in vivo stimulation of stem-cell recovery and hematopoietic regeneration following 5-fluorouracil treatment of mice. *Proc Natl Acad Sci USA.* **84**, 7134–8.

Moreb J, Zucali JR, Gross MA and Weiner RS (1989). Protective effects of IL-1 on human hematopoietic progenitor cells treated in vitro with 4-hydroperoxycyclophosphamide. *J Immunol.* **142**, 1937–42.

Morikage T, Mizushima Y, Sakamoto K and Yano S (1990). Prevention of fatal infections by recombinant human interleukin 1 alpha in normal and anticancer drug-treated mice. *Cancer Res.* **50**, 2099–2104.

Mortensen RF, Shapiro J, Lin B-, Douches S and Neta R. (1988). Interaction of recombinant IL-1 and recombinant tumor necrosis factor in the induction of mouse acute phase proteins. *J Immunol.* **140**, 2260–6.

Moser R, Schleiffenbaum B, Groscurth P and Fehr J (1989). Interleukin-1 and tumor necrosis factor stimulate human vascular endothelial cells to promote transendothelial neutrophil passage. *J Clin Invest.* **83**, 444–55.

Nakamura S, Minami A, Fujimoto K and Kojima T (1989). Combination effect of recombinant human interleukin-1 alpha with antimicrobial agents. *Antimicrob Agents Chemother.* **33**, 1804–10.

Nakamura S, Kashimoto S, Kajikawa F and Nakata K (1991). Combination effect of recombinant human interleukin 1 alpha with antitumor drugs on syngeneic tumors in mice. *Cancer Res.* **51**, 215–21.

Nawroth PP, Bank I, Handley D *et al.* (1986). Tumor necrosis factor/cachectin interacts with endothelial cell receptors to induce release of interleukin 1. *J Exp Med.* **163**, 1363–99.

Neta R (1990). Radioprotection and therapy of radiation injury with cytokines. *Prog Clin Biol Res.* **352**, 471–8.

Numerof RP, Aronson FR, and Mier JW (1988). IL-2 stimulates the production of IL–1α and IL-1β by human peripheral blood mononuclear cells. *J Immunol.* **141**, 4250–7.

Okusawa S, Gelfand JA, Ikejima T *et al.* (1988). IL-1 induces a shock like state in rabbits. Synergism with tumor necrosis factor and the effect of cyclooxygenase inhibition. *J Clin Invest.* **81**, 1162–72.

Oster W, Cicco NA, Klein H *et al.* (1989). Participation of the cytokines interleukin 6, tumor necrosis factor-alpha, and interleukin 1-beta secreted by acute myelogenous leukemia blasts in autocrine and paracrine leukemia growth control. *J Clin Invest.* **84**, 451–457.

Ridgway D, Borzy MS and Bagby GC (1988). Granulocyte macrophage colony stimulating activity production by cultured human thymic non-lymphoid cells is regulated by endogenous interleukin-1. *Blood.* **72**, 1230–6.

Roll JT, Young KM, Kurtz RS and Czuprynski CJ (1990). Human rTNF alpha augments anti-bacterial resistance in mice: potentiation of its effects by recombinant human rIL-1 alpha. *Immunology.* **69**, 316–22.

Salmon SE and Liu R (1989). Effects of granulocyte-macrophage colony-stimulating factor on in vitro growth of human solid tumors. *J Clin Oncol.* **7**, 1346–50.

Sapolsky R, Rivier C, Yamamoto G *et al.* (1987). Interleukin-1 stimulates the secretion of hypothalamic corticotropin-releasing factor. *Science.* **238**, 522–4.

Schwartz GN, MacVittie TJ, Vigneulle RM *et al.* (1987). Enhanced hematopoietic recovery in irradiated mice pretreated with interleukin-1 (IL-1). *Immunopharmacol Immunotoxicol.* **9**, 371–89.

Seelentag W, Mermod J-J and Vassalli P (1989). Interleukin 1 and tumor necrosis factor-α additively increase the levels of granulocyte-macrophage and granulocyte colony- stimulating factor (CSF) mRNA in human fibroblasts. *Eur J Immunol.* **19**, 209–12.

Segal GM and Bagby GC (1988). Vascular endothelial cells and hematopoietic regulation. *Int J Cell Cloning*. **6**, 306–312.

Segal GM, McCall E and Bagby GC (1988). The erythroid burst promoting activity produced by interleukin-1 stimulated endothelial cells is granulocyte macrophage colony stimulating factor. *Blood.* **72**, 1364–7.

Semenza GL, Traystman MD, Gearhart JD and Antonarakis SE (1989). Polycythemia in transgenic mice expressing the human erythropoietin gene. *Proc Natl Acad Sci USA.* **86**, 2301–5.

Silver GM, Gamelli RL, O'Reilly M and Hebert JC (1990). The effect of interleukin-1 alpha on survival in a murine model of burn wound sepsis. *Arch Surg.* **125**, 922–5.

Sims JE, March CJ, Cosman D *et al.* (1988). cDNA expression cloning of the IL-1 receptor, a member of the immunoglobulin superfamily. *Science.* **241**, 585–589.

Sisson SD and Dinarello CA (1988). Production of interleukin-1a, interleukin-1 and tumor necrosis factor by human mononuclear cells stimulated with granulocyte-macrophage colony-stimulating factor. *Blood.* **72**, 1368–74.

Stohlman FJR, Rath CE and Rose JC (1954). Evidence for a humoral regulation of erythropoiesis: studies on a patient with polycythemia secondary to regional hypoxia. *Blood.* **9**, 721–33.

Stork, L, Barczuk L, Kissinger M and Robinson W (1989). Interleukin-1 accelerates murine granulocyte recovery following treatment with cyclophosphamide. *Blood.* **73**, 938–44.

Stork LC, Peterson VM, Rundus CH and Robinson WA (1988). Interleukin-1 enhances murine granulopoiesis in vivo. *Exp Hematol.* **16**, 163–7.

Suematsu S, Hibi M, Sugita T *et al.* (1990). Interleukin 6 (IL-6) and its receptor (IL-6R) in myeloma/plasmacytoma. *Curr Top Microbiol. Immunol.* **166**, 13–22.

van der Meer JW, Rubin RH, Pasternack M *et al.* (1989a). The in vivo and in vitro effects of interleukin-1 and tumor necrosis factor on murine cytomegalovirus infection. *Biotherapy.* **1**, 227–31.

van der Meer JWM, Helle M and Aarden L (1989b). Comparison of the effects of recombinant interleukin 6 and recombinant interleukin 1 on nonspecific resistance to infection. *Eur. J Immunol.* **19**, 413–16.

Van't Wout JW, van der Meer JWM, Barza M and Dinarello CA (1988). Protection of neutropenic mice from lethal Candida albicans infection by recombinant interleukin 1. *Eur J Immunol.* **18**,1143–6.

Wakabayashi G, Gelfand JA, Burke JF *et al.* (1991). A specific receptor antagonist for interleukin 1 prevents Escherichia coli-induced shock in rabbits. *FASEB J.* **5**, 338–43.

Warner SJC, Auger KR and Libby P (1987). Interleukin-1 induces interleukin-1 II. Recombinant human interleukin-1 induces interleukin-1 production by adult human vascular endothelial cells. *J Immunol.* **139**, 1911–17.

Webb AC, Collins KL, Auron PE *et al.* (1986). Interleukin-1 gene (IL1) assigned to long arm of human chromosome 2. *Lymphokine Res.* **5**, 77.

White CW and Ghezzi P (1989). Protection against pulmonary oxygen toxicity by interleukin-1 and tumor necrosis factor: role of antioxidant enzymes and effect of cyclooxygenase inhibitors. *Biotherapy.* **1**, 361–7.

Wu SG and Miyamoto T (1990). Radioprotection of the intestinal crypts of mice by recombinant human interleukin-1 alpha. *Radiat Res.* **123**, 112–15.

Zhan YF, Stanley ER and Cheers C (1991). Prophylaxis or treatment of experimental brucellosis with interleukin-1. *Infect Immun.* **59**, 1790–4.

Zsebo KM, Yuschenkoff V, Schulter S *et al.* (1988). Vascular endothelial cells and granulopoiesis: Interleukin-1 stimulates release of G-CSF and GM-CSF. *Blood.* **71**, 99–103.

Zucali JR, Dinarello CA, Oblon DJ, Gross MA, Anderson L and Weiner RS (1986). Interleukin-1 stimulates fibroblasts to produce granulocyte-macrophage colony stimulating activity and prostaglandin E2. *J Clin Invest.* **77**, 1857–63.

6

INTERLEUKIN-2

P. M. SONDEL

INTRODUCTION

Interleukin-2 (IL-2) has no known antiproliferative influence on the tumours that have shown responses to it, distinguishing it from other clinical modalities used for cancer therapy. The action of IL-2 appears to be mediated through the cells of the immune system that respond to IL-2 (Borden and Sondel, 1990). Some of these cellular responses to IL-2 can have readily measurable, yet still poorly characterized, antitumour effects. Following the initial report of clinical benefit for some cancer patients receiving IL-2 (Rosenberg et al., 1985), an international effort has further tested the clinical utility of this molecule. Many patients have shown dramatic tumour regressions induced by IL-2-based therapy. Nevertheless, most patients who have been treated with regimens containing IL-2 have not shown evidence of antitumour benefit. Preclinical models have shown a variety of variables that can influence the efficacy of IL-2 in inducing tumour destruction in vivo by activating cellular immune responses (Kedar et al., 1989). Improvements in the clinical efficacy of IL-2 will probably require better control of these clinical variables to enable effective tumour control by cellular immune mechanisms.

CELLULAR IMMUNE RESPONSES TO MALIGNANT CELLS

Clinical testing of IL-2 has been based, in part, on somewhat anecdotal observations over the past century, suggesting that immunological responses may have antitumour effects. These clinical observations stimulated well focused animal experimentation, which proved that cellular immune responses can prevent the growth or spread of certain experimentally induced or transplanted neoplasms. These models have shown that T lymphocytes, natural killer (NK) lymphocytes, B lymphocytes and the antibodies they produce, monocytes and the cytokines secreted by all of these cells can be involved in immune control of murine tumours. In several models the roles of the T lymphocytes and NK lymphocytes have been most important (Mule *et al.*, 1987).

Immune responses by T lymphocytes are initiated by specific recognition of antigenic peptides that are presented by major histocompatibility complex (MHC) molecules. For T cell responses to certain murine tumours, the genetically rearranged α/β T cell receptor complex recognizes MHC-presented viral peptides of the oncogenic virus expressed by the murine tumour cells (Cheever *et al.*, 1986; Klarnet *et al*, 1989). Somewhat analogous recognition of autologous human tumours has been described in certain in vitro analyses. However, it has been difficult to demonstrate MHC-restricted specific recognition of many human tumours, and even for those tumours that are well recognized by T cells, the specific 'tumour peptides' have been difficult to identify. It remains possible that some human tumours might not express MHC-presented tumour-specific peptides that can be readily recognized by autologous T lymphocytes.

In contrast, NK lymphocytes can bind to and destroy a variety of transformed, virally infected, and certain neoplastic tissues in vitro (Robertson and Ritz, 1990). Several cell surface adhesion molecules are involved in NK recognition of target tissues; this NK-mediated recognition does not show the fine specificity characteristic of T cell recognition (Phillips and Lanier, 1986; Whiteside and Herberman, 1989). Natural killer cells appear to recognize a broad variety of tissues in a somewhat non-specific way; they do not appear to use a T-cell-like genetically recombined receptor mechanism. Thus, activated NK cells can destroy normal tissues as well as transformed or neoplastic ones (Sondel *et al.*, 1986). Despite this 'non-specificity' certain murine models have utilized endogenous, activated or transplanted NK cells to prevent growth of experimental tumours.

MOLECULAR COMMUNICATION BETWEEN IMMUNE CELLS

An intact immune response involves multiple complex cellular interactions. The immune system uses a variety of molecules to enable communication between the different cellular components of the immune response. These molecules, designated 'interleukins', allow immunoregulatory communication (Smith *et al.*, 1980). One of these molecules is interleukin-2, a glycoprotein with a relative molecular mass of 15 kDa, which is involved in virtually all cellular immune responses (Smith *et al.*, 1980). IL-2 is a major controlling element in the activation, proliferation, in vivo expansion and function of both T cells and NK cells.

THE BIOLOGY OF INTERLEUKIN-2

Once T cells have used their T cell receptor to recognize MHC-presented antigen, these cells are activated to further differentiate (Smith, 1988). Following interaction with monocytes or macrophages, helper T cells then release interleukin 2, which stimulates further expansion of helper T cell populations, and activates other populations of T cells, as well as NK cells, B cells, and monocytes (Smith, 1988).

The cells of the immune system recognize IL-2 through a membrane–IL-2 receptor complex. This IL-2 receptor consists of either a moderate affinity 70 kD α chain, or a high affinity bimolecular complex consisting of the β chain and a 55 kDa α chain (Waldman, 1989). The recognition and response to IL-2 by the IL-2 receptor probably involves additional molecular components of the IL-2 receptor complex (Voss *et al.*, 1990). This complex membrane receptor mechanism could potentially regulate the differential activation of distinct subpopulations of lymphocytes, in a response modulated by the IL-2 concentration, and the prior activation state of the IL-2 responsive cells.

Once the membrane–IL-2 receptor complex has been triggered by IL-2, transmembrane signalling events induce intracellular changes that are rapidly detectable at the nuclear level by alterations in mRNA synthesis. The IL-2-responsive lymphocytes proliferate, differentiate, and make a variety of molecules involved in these cellular reactions. Important molecules in this response are those molecules used by effector lymphocytes to destroy target tissue (Borden and Sondel, 1990).

CLINICAL POTENTIAL OF IL-2

As IL-2 is a critical component of virtually any immune response, augmentation or inhibition of IL-2 action could potentially be utilized in a variety of clinical conditions influenced by the immune system. Immune deficiency disorders, including those associated with inherited defects in IL-2 production or response mechanisms, might be circumvented by clinical provision of exogenous IL-2 (Pahwa *et al.*, 1989). Future applications could involve provision of IL-2 to enhance ongoing cellular immune responses to severe infection, or to enhance the efficacy of active immunization with immunoprotective vaccination therapies. In contrast, deleterious immune responses, such as a variety of autoimmune disorders, or the rejection of organ allografts, might be blunted by inhibiting the action of IL-2. Antibodies directed against IL-2 itself, against the IL-2 receptor, or potent toxins conjugated to IL-2 molecules able to bind to immune cells through the IL-2 receptor complex, are all being investigated as immunosuppressive treatments (Waldman, 1989). These 'immunosuppressive' approaches might also be useful in treating certain neoplasms that express IL-2 receptors (such as T cell leukaemias and lymphomas). However, these possibilities are all distinct from the use of IL-2 to augment cellular immune responses that may have a direct in vivo antitumour effect. It is this latter approach that has been the focus of most clinical testing with IL-2.

PRECLINICAL TESTING OF IL-2 IN ANIMAL MODELS

In vivo treatment with IL-2 has proceeded in a number of species. Results from a myriad of murine in vivo models have been of great importance in the design of many clinical trials. Early murine studies suggested IL-2 might best activate immune cells that were already triggered by antigen recognition to express their membrane IL-2 receptors (Smith et al., 1980). In this way, IL-2 might be effective in augmenting the transfer of tumour-specific T lymphocytes that could recognize MHC-presented 'tumour-specific peptides' on experimentally induced murine tumours. IL-2 was of clear benefit in models testing this experimental situation (Cheever et al., 1986). However, and somewhat unexpectedly, infusion of IL-2 was also of benefit in control of 'non-immunogenic' murine tumours where tumour-specific T cell responses could not be identified (Mule et al., 1987). The mechanism of action of IL-2 in the 'non-immunogenic' setting appeared to be primarily through activated NK cells. These many murine studies documented that IL-2 was usually more effective for certain tumours recognized specifically by T cells, was more protective when given to animals bearing only microscopic amounts of tumour, and required immune cells (either T or NK) capable of responding to the IL-2 to mediate tumour destruction (Mule et al., 1987). Infusion of in vitro IL-2-activated lymphocytes, designated lymphokine activated killer (LAK) cells, could often augment the antitumour efficacy of IL-2, but these exogenous lymphocytes were not essential. More dramatic antitumour effects were often seen with higher doses of IL-2. Pharmacokinetic analyses of IL-2 showed a rapid half-life of i.v. IL-2 given as a rapid bolus injection. The need for effective molecular interaction of IL-2 with its receptor, and the short half-life of IL-2, suggested that approaches that prolong an effective IL-2 level might have a greater immune activating effect. Finally, and somewhat unexpectedly, in the initial murine studies significant immune-mediated toxicity was noted with higher doses of IL-2 (Ettinghausen *et al.*, 1988). These toxicities appeared to reflect the direct cell-mediated injury by IL-2-activated lymphocytes against certain normal tissues, as well as the release by these cells of cytokines and other biologically active, potentially toxic molecules (such as tumour necrosis factor).

Most of the conclusions from murine models have been predictive of the clinical results that have now been obtained in clinical studies treating cancer patients with recombinant IL-2. To use IL-2 as more effective clinical immunotherapy, it will be necessary to take advantage of the antitumour mechanisms induced by IL-2 while preventing the toxicities.

EVALUATION OF HUMAN RECOMBINANT IL-2 AS CANCER THERAPY

Clinical trials with IL-2 alone or with in vitro IL-2-activated LAK infusions

Innovative clinical research using IL-2, by Rosenberg and colleagues from the National Cancer Institute, demonstrated that an immunological approach aimed at activating endogenous host immune mechanisms could clearly and reproducibly induce antitumour effects in some patients with refractory malignancies (Rosenberg *et al.*, 1987). Some patients with melanoma and renal cell carcinoma could show complete or partial tumour shrinkage in response to IL-2-based therapy. Unfortunately, only a minority of patients experience the desired tumour shrinkage. Most of these responses are transient, but occasional patients show durable antitumour effects lasting several years.

Somewhat comparable results have been generated at cancer centres world-wide, using the same regimen developed at the National Cancer Institute (Fisher *et al.*, 1988; Parkinson, 1988; Dutcher *et al.*, 1989; Hawkins, 1989), as well as several other regimens utilizing IL-2 alone or with IL-2-activated LAK cell infusions (West *et al.*, 1987; Eberlein *et al.*, 1988; Sosman *et al.*, 1988a, b; Paciucci *et al.*, 1989). Even though the antitumour response rates from the National Cancer Institute were somewhat higher than those reported by others using similar or different IL-2 regimens, the aggregate testing proved that some melanoma and renal cell carcinoma patients could respond to IL-2 utilizing a variety of regimens.

Despite a vast array of clinical approaches using IL-2, most published results are consistent with the following general conclusions:

1. IL-2 induces immune system activation, in a dose-dependent way, in virtually all cancer patients receiving this treatment. In vivo activation by IL-2 is characterized by rebound lymphocytosis following IL-2 treatment, activation of endogenous NK cells (detected by flow cytometry and their ability to mediate LAK activity in vitro), and a variety of other well described immunological changes that measure modification of T cell and NK function (Hank et al., 1988; Thompson et al., 1988; Sondel et al., 1989; Urba et al., 1990).

2. The toxicities of IL-2 are dose-dependent, immune-mediated, and reproducible (Sosman et al., 1988a,b; Dutcher et al., 1989). These toxicities are rapidly reversible and therefore can be clinically managed by appropriate supportive therapy, stopping the IL-2 treatment if toxicities become severe and targeting the dose of IL-2 to be utilized to the level of toxicity appropriate for the clinical situation.

3. The infusion > 10^{10} in vitro activated LAK cells intravenously might, in certain situations, slightly increase the likelihood of antitumour responses when added to IL-2 alone, although this remains uncertain. However, the infusion of LAK cells can add substantially to the complexity and cost of administering IL-2-based therapy; and can add to the toxicity of a relatively well tolerated IL-2 regimen (Albertini et al., 1990).

4. None of the many immunological parameters clearly influenced by IL-2 have been of great prospective utility in predicting toxicity or antitumour effects of IL-2-based therapy. Certain parameters have shown statistically significant correlations with antitumour response or toxicity (i.e. DR expression on tumours, and serum IL-2 receptor levels). These values have not yet been useful in making clinical decisions for individual patients (Bogner et al., 1991).

5. Despite the striking antitumour responses seen in some patients, most patients do not show any measurable objective clinical benefit in response to IL-2, even though most patients experience some degree of IL-2 induced toxicity. Improvements in IL-2-based therapies are clearly needed.

Testing designed to improve single agent treatment with IL-2

Several opportunities might enable improved treatment involving single agent IL-2 therapy. First, is the evaluation of systemic IL-2 for patients in remission, bearing only microscopic amounts of residual tumour. Preclinical studies suggest greater tumour protection might be provided by this approach (Cheever et al., 1986; Mule et al., 1987; Kedar et al., 1989); however, which dose, delivery method and schedule to use in adjuvant clinical testing remains unresolved. Secondly, enhanced antitumour effects can be obtained experimentally when IL-2 is injected locally into the tumour itself. Local injection of IL-2 (with or without LAK cells) has shown some antitumour responses in treatment of certain clinical malignancies, including CNS neoplasms, head and neck tumours, and hepatic carcinoma (Nitta *et al.*, 1990). Of importance in the subsequent development of this concept will be the testing of the hypothesis that IL-2 administration in a local tumour site could potentially augment systemic antitumour immune mechanisms able to destroy disseminated micrometastases. 'Gene therapy' approaches in which IL-2 is produced at the tumour site by using tumour cells transfected to express IL-2 are now being proposed to more effectively provide IL-2 at an immunizing tumour site. Another approach might better clarify those pretreatment variables that are predictive of a given patient showing tumour shrinkage or profound toxicity to IL-2-based therapy. Identification of such parameters could allow selection of patients most likely to benefit from IL-2 and identify those less likely to respond to IL-2 so they could receive other approaches or other combinations. Finally, as the molecular mechanisms of IL-2-induced toxicity are better identified (such as tumour necrosis factor release), some of their immune-mediated toxicity might potentially be 'blocked' by agents that do not necessarily eliminate the antitumour immune effects. Clinical testing of these principles could allow prolonged IL-2 activation of antitumour mechanisms while ameliorating some of the indirect toxicities of IL-2 (such as hypotension associated with vasodilation).

IL-2 in combination with other cancer treatments

Immunotherapeutic approaches can be augmented in murine models when combined with certain other cytokines (such as interferons and tumour necrosis factor), radiation therapy and chemotherapy. Many antitumour mechanisms may be at work in such combinations. Clinical testing of some of these many approaches is underway and multiple clinical variables require careful scrutiny to evaluate the results of these treatments objectively (Mitchell *et al.*, 1988; Rosenberg *et al.*, 1988a,b; Kedar *et al.*, 1989).

Interleukin-2 and tumour-specific immune recognition

IL-2-based clinical testing has recently evaluated the combination of IL-2 plus tumour infiltrating lymphocytes (Rosenberg *et al.*, 1988b). In certain murine models, tumour-specific T lymphocytes can be propagated in vitro from a variety of in vivo sources, including those lymphocytes found to be infiltrating the tumour itself. More recent in vitro analyses of human lymphocytes have shown that tumour-specific T lymphocytes that appear to be recognizing autologous tumour in a MHC-restricted way, can occasionally recognize and destroy autologous melanoma in certain patients. These autologous, tumour-specific, T lymphocytes have been found in peripheral blood (Mukherji et al., 1989) as well as in the tumour infiltrating lymphocyte (TIL) population for some patients. These tumour-specific T lymphocytes might have therapeutic advantages over LAK cells when combined with IL-2, if the murine models are predictive. However, in vitro analyses of expanded TIL specimens from many patients with melanoma, and most patients with other malignancies, show effector cell function more consistent with the non-MHC-restricted LAK phenomenon, than that of tumour specific MHC-restricted T lymphocytes. One advantage of tumour-specific T lymphocytes is reflected by the ability of these T cells (at least from some patients) to show some degree of preferential ability to infiltrate tumour sites in vivo. Unfortunately, many patients whose tumours have been biopsied in order to generate therapeutic TIL populations have shown progressive tumour growth prior to being able to receive these in vitro expanded cells (and thus did not get TIL treatment), were not able to generate sufficient growth of the TIL cultures in vitro to enable their use as therapy, or did not generate tumour-specific T lymphocytes (suggesting that, for them, the IL-2 plus TIL therapy was no different than IL-2 plus LAK therapy, which would have been more simple). Nevertheless, for certain melanoma patients, and possibly other patients, the potential for improved in vitro sensitization, selection, and expansion of bulk cultures of tumour-specific T lymphocytes (Barnd et al., 1989) may offer an added dimension for IL-2 treatment, taking advantage of tumour-specific recognition by these T cells.

Currently, IL-2 plus TIL approaches are moving in three separate directions. One approach involves insertion of potentially therapeutic genes into the TIL populations that show tumour-specific reactivities. The products of such transplanted genes (such as tumour necrosis factor) could potentially enable more effective tumour destruction by the tumour-specific T cells (Rosenberg et al., 1990), provided that they selectively get to the tumour site. Secondly, current improvements in in vitro techniques are now allowing identification of individual T cell clones, with selection for clones that show relative degrees of tumour specificity. Expansion of larger numbers of such preselected clones to allow clinical transfer may provide a dimension for specific immunological therapy not possible with non-cloned heterogeneous lymphocyte cultures (Sosman et al., 1990). Finally, the demonstration of tumour-specific T cell reactivity to some human tumours, supports the important hypothesis that these T cells are recognizing peptides presented by the MHC that might be shared between histologically similar allogeneic tumours (Crowley *et al.*, 1990). If this is the case, TIL research currently underway might enable characterization of those tumour-specific peptides to allow generation of clinically effective active immunization vaccination approaches.

IL-2 combined with tumour reactive antibodies

Following a decade of clinical research, a number of clinical grade monoclonal antibodies have been selected and show a relative degree of tumour selectivity in their ability to recognize certain human tumours better than normal human tissues. These antibodies may potentially bring drugs or toxins directly to the tumour site. Certain of these antibodies are recognized by lymphocytes and other effector cells that bear Fc receptors and thus mediate antibody-directed cellular cytotoxicity (ADCC) of tumour cells. To be effective in vivo, cells able to mediate ADCC must be well activated; in vivo therapy with IL-2 can clearly accomplish this (Hank *et al.*, 1990). Molecular engineering approaches are now improving the quality of antibody molecules for clinical testing; a family of tumour-selective human–mouse chimeric antibodies is now entering clinical testing and further molecular engineering and selection approaches are likely to generate molecules able to better home and selectively recognize tumour in vivo. Combining those antibodies able to mediate ADCC with in vivo effector cell activation utilizing IL-2 is now being tested in a variety of ongoing clinical trials.

This IL-2 antibody approach could be combined with in vivo infusion of other cytokines, such as M-CSF or GM-CSF, to potentiate the ability of myeloid and monocytoid cells to mediate in vivo ADCC. These cytokines could potentially be combined with a cocktail of distinct tumour-reactive genetically engineered monoclonal antibodies, to enable a multifaceted attack against residual tumour cells. If such an approach were used in the adjuvant setting it may be a means to the selective eradication of residual neoplastic disease. Initiation of such complex clinical approaches, dependent upon recombinant technology for a variety of components, requires a stepwise approach to combining these agents, which is now being initiated.

OVERVIEW

IL-2 can activate antitumour immune mechanisms directly within certain cancer patients. Some patients with large tumours have shown tumour shrinkage after IL-2 treatment even though murine studies indicated that treatment of bulky tumours (especially if non-immunogenic) might not be effective with single-agent IL-2 therapy. On-going studies are better characterizing the detailed interactions of T cells and NK cells with human neoplasms. Tumour-specific antigenic peptides and tumour-selective antibody reagents are being characterized or generated through molecular engineering approaches. These advances should make it possible to combine these multiple innovative immunological approaches together with more conventional antitumour therapies. Clinical studies of these combinations will test the possibility of adding effective immunological therapy to standard clinical cancer care. Data already obtained from clinical trials of IL-2 indicate that in vivo activation of effector cell mechanisms in a reproducible, controlled and dose-dependent manner with IL-2 may play an important role in the future of these combined immunotherapeutic approaches.

ACKNOWLEDGEMENTS

The research summarized in this chapter reflects experiences of multiple laboratory and clinical research teams world-wide, yet this review does not attempt a comprehensive citation of the massive body of literature in this expanding field. Work cited from our research team is supported by NIH Grants CA-32685, RR-03186, CM-87290, CA-53441, CA-20432, NIH support to the UW Comprehensive Cancer Center, and American Cancer Society Grant CH-237. Grateful thanks are given to J. A. Hank who has been involved in all aspects of these studies, and to M. Pankratz and J. Anderson for preparation of this chapter.

REFERENCES

Albertini MA, Sosman JA, Hank JA et al. (1990). The influence of autologous lymphokine activated killer cell infusions on the toxicity and antitumour effect of repetitive cycles of interleukin 2. *Cancer.* **66**, 2457–64.
Barnd DL, Lan MS, Metzgar RS and Finn OJ (1989). Specific major histocompatibility complex – unrestricted recognition of tumour-associated mucins by human cytotoxic T cells. *Proc Natl Acad Sci (USA).* **86**, 7159–63.
Bogner MP, Voss SD, Bechhofer R et al. (1991). Dose response to IL-2 therapy and correlations with clinical toxicity and surface TAC expression on post-therapy peripheral blood lymphocytes (submitted).
Borden EC and Sondel PM (1990). Lymphokines and cytokines as cancer treatment: immunotherapy realized. *Cancer.* **65**, 800–14.

P. M. SONDEL

Cheever MA, Thompson DB, Klarnet JP and Greenberg PD (1986). Antigen-driven long-term cultured T cells proliferate in vivo, distribute widely, mediate specific tumour therapy and persist long-term as functional memory T cells. *J Exp Med.* 163, 1100–12.

Crowley NJ, Slingluff CL, Darrow TL and Seigler HF (1990). Generation of autologous melanoma specific cytotoxic T-cells using HLA-A2-matched allogeneic melanomas. *Cancer Res.* 50, 492–8.

Dutcher JP, Creekmore SP, Weiss GR *et al.* (1989). A phase II study of interleukin 2 and lymphokine-activated killer cells in patients with metastatic malignant melanoma. *J Clin Oncol.* 7, 477–85.

Eberlein TJ, Schoof DD, Jung S *et al.* (1988). A new regimen of interleukin 2 and lymphokine activated killer cells: Efficacy without significant toxicity. *Arch Int Med.* 148, 2571–6.

Ettinghausen SE, Puri RK and Rosenberg SA (1988). Increased vascular permeability in organs mediated by systemic administration of lymphokine activated killer cells and recombinant interleukin 2 in mice. *J Natl Cancer Inst.* 80, 177–88.

Fisher RI, Coltman CA, Doroshow JH *et al.* (1988). Metastatic renal cancer treated with interleukin 2 and lymphokine activated killer cells. *Ann. Int Med.* 108, 518–23.

Hank JA, Kohler PC, Hillman GH *et al.* (1988). Interleukin 2 (IL-2) dependent human lymphokine activated killer (LAK) cells generated in vivo during administration of human recombinant IL-2. *Cancer Res.* 48, 1965–71.

Hank JA, Robinson RR, Surfus J *et al.* (1990). Augmentation of antibody dependent cell mediated cytotoxicity following in vivo therapy with recombinant interleukin-2. *Cancer Res.* 50, 5234–9.

Hawkins MJ (1989). IL-2/LAK: Current status and possible future directions. *Principals and Practice of Oncology: Updates.* 3(8), 1–14.

Kedar E, Ben-Aziz R, Epstein E and Leshem B (1989). Chemo-immunotherapy of murine tumours using IL-2 and cyclophosphamide. *Cancer Immunol Immunother.* 29, 74–8.

Klarnet JP, Kern DE, Okuno K *et al.* (1989). FBL-reactive Lyt-2+ cytotoxic and L3T4+ helper T lymphocytes recognize distinct F-MuLV-encoded antigens. *J Exp Med.* 169, 457–67.

Mitchell MS, Kempf RA, Harel W *et al.* (1988). Effectiveness and tolerability of low dose cyclophosphamide and low dose intravenous interleukin 2 in disseminated melanoma. *J Clin Oncol.* 6, 409–24.

Mukherji B, Guha A, Chakraborty N *et al.* (1989). Clonal analysis of cytotoxic and regulatory T-cell responses against human melanoma. *J Exp Med.* 169, 1961–79.

Mule JJ, Yang JC, Lafreniere R, Shu S and Rosenberg SA (1987). Identification of cellular mechanisms operational in vivo during the regression of established pulmonary metastases by the systemic administration of high dose recombinant interleukin 2. *J Immunol.* 139, 285–295.

88

Nitta T, Sato K, Yagita H, Okumura K and Ishii S (1990). Preliminary trial of specifictargeting therapy against malignant glioma. *Lancet*. **i**, 368–71.

Paciucci PA, Holland JF, Ryder JS *et al*. (1989). Immunotherapy with interleukin 2 by constant infusion with and without adoptive cell transfer and with weekly doxorubicin. *Cancer Treat Rev*. **16 (Suppl. A)**, 67–81.

Pahwa R, Chatila T, Pahwa S *et al*. (1989). Recombinant interleukin 2 therapy in severe combined immunodeficiency disease. *Proc Natl Acad Sci (USA)*. **86**, 5069–73.

Parkinson DR (1988). Interleukin 2 in cancer therapy. *Sem in Oncol*. **15 (6 Suppl.)**, 10–26.

Phillips JH and Lanier LL (1986). Dissection of the lymphokine–activated killer phenomenon. Relative contribution of peripheral blood natural killer cells and T lymphocytes to cytolysis. *J Exp Med*. **164**, 814–25.

Robertson MJ and Ritz J (1990). Biology and clinical relevance of human natural killer cells. *Blood*. **76**, 2421–30.

Rosenberg SA, Lotze MT, Muul LM *et al*. (1985). Observations on the systemic administration of autologous lymphokine-activated killer cells and recombinant interleukin 2 to patients with metastatic cancer. *New Engl J Med*. **313**, 1485–92.

Rosenberg SA, Lotze MT, Muul LM *et al*. (1987). A progress report on the treatment of 157 patients with advanced cancer using lymphokine activated killer cells and interleukin 2 or high dose interleukin 2 alone. *New Engl J Med*. **316**, 889–97.

Rosenberg SA, Lotze MT and Mule JJ (1988a). New approaches to the immunotherapy of cancer using interleukin 2. *Annals Inter Med*. **B**, 853–64.

Rosenberg SA, Packard B, Aebersold P *et al*. (1988b). Use of tumour-infiltrating lymphocytes and interleukin-2 in the immunotherapy of patients with metastatic melanoma. *New Engl J Med*. **319**, 1676–80.

Rosenberg SA, Aebersold P, Cornetta K *et al*. (1990). Gene transfer into humans – Immunotherapy of patients with advanced melanoma using tumour infiltrating lymphocytes modified by retroviral gene translocation. *New Engl J Med*. **323**, 570–8.

Smith KA (1988). Interleukin 2: Inception, impact, and implications. *Science*. **240**, 1169–76.

Smith KA, Lachmann LB, Oppenheim JJ and Favata MF (1980). The functional relationship of the interleukins. *J Exp Med*. **151**, 1551–6.

Sondel PM, Hank JA, Kohler PC *et al*. (1986). Destruction of autologous human lymphocytes by interleukin 2-activated cytotoxic cells. *J Immunol*. **137**, 502–11.

Sondel PM, Hank JA, Kohler C *et al*. (1989). The cellular immunotherapy of cancer: Current and potential uses of interleukin-2. *Criti Rev Oncology/ Hematology*. **9**, 125–47.

Sosman JA, Kohler PC, Hank JA *et al*. (1988a). Repetitive weekly cycles of recombinant human interleukin 2: Responses of renal carcinoma with acceptable toxicity. *J Natl Cancer Inst*. **80**, 60–63.

Sosman JA, Kohler PC, Hank JA *et al.* (1988b). Repetitive weekly cycles of interleukin 2. II. Clinical and immunologic effects of dose, schedule, and addition of indomethacin. *J Natl Cancer Inst.* **80**, 1451–61.

Sosman JA, Oettel K, Smith SD *et al.* (1990). Specific recognition of human leukemic cells by allogeneic T cells: II. Evidence for HLA-D restricted unique determinants on leukemic cells which are cross-reactive with determinants present on unrelated non-leukemic cells. *Blood.* **75**, 2005–16.

Thompson JA, Lee DJ, Lindgren CG *et al.* (1988). Influence of dose and duration of infusion of interleukin 2 on toxicity and immunomodulation. *J Clin Oncol.* **6**, 669–78.

Urba WJ, Steis RS, Longo D *et al.* (1990). Immunomodulatory properties and toxicity of interleukin 2 in patients with cancer. *Cancer Res.* **50**, 185–92.

Voss SD, Robb RJ, Weil-Hillman G *et al.* (1990). Increased expression of the IL-2 receptor β chain (p70) on CD56+ NK cells following in vivo IL-2 therapy: p70 expression does not alone predict the level of intermediate-affinity IL-2 binding. *J Exp Med.* **172**, 1101–14.

Waldmann TR (1989). The multi-subunit interleukin 2 receptor. *Ann Rev Biochem.* **58**, 875–911.

West WH, Tauer KW, Yannelli JR *et al.* (1987). Constant infusion recombinant interleukin 2 in adoptive immunotherapy of cancer. *New Engl J Med.* **316**, 898–905.

Whiteside TL and Herberman RB (1989). The role of natural killer cells in human disease. *Clin Immunol Immunopath.* **53**, 1–23.

7

INTERLEUKIN-3

A. GANSER, O. G. OTTMANN and D. HOELZER

INTRODUCTION

The control mechanisms governing the maintainance of haemopoiesis throughout all stages of differentiation are complex and only fragmentarily understood. They form a regulatory network that involves stromal cell signals, cell adhesion molecules and matrix proteins. Furthermore, the potential role of such soluble factors as haemopoietic growth regulators has been underscored by several recent studies.

The lymphokine interleukin-3 (IL-3) is one member of a family of haemopoietic growth factors known as colony-stimulating factors (CSF) (Yang and Clark, 1989). These glycoproteins not only support the survival, proliferation and differentiation of various types of haemopoietic progenitors, but also modulate the functional activity of mature blood cells. Several of these CSFs, e.g. erythropoietin (EPO), granulocyte-CSF (G-CSF) or macrophage-CSF (M-CSF), are relatively cell-type- and/or stage-specific in their actions. Conversely, IL-3 was found from the outset to possess a considerably broader spectrum of activities, while the activity of granulocyte–macrophage CSF (GM-CSF) lies in between the multilineage activity of IL-3 and those of the lineage-restricted CSFs (Morstyn and Burgess, 1988).

The biological feature central to the interest in IL-3 is this molecule's apparent involvement in the growth regulation of primitive pluripotent haemopoietic progenitor cells, possibly including those that retain self-renewal capacity (Valent et al., 1990). These latter activities have been difficult to study experimentally, and the precise role of IL-3 in physiological regulation of myelopoiesis has not yet been ascertained. Nevertheless, there is substantial interest in the therapeutic application of IL-3 in the treatment of primary or drug-induced cytopenias, in bone marrow transplantation and as an agent capable of enhancing overall host defence (Valent *et al.*, 1990; Garnick and O'Reilly, 1989).

BIOLOGICAL PROPERTIES OF IL-3

Identification of IL-3

The concept that IL-3 functions as a regulator of early lympho-haemopoietic development originated from studies in the murine system. In experiments examining early T cell differentiation, a factor was identified that induced the expression of the T-cell-associated enzyme 20-alpha-hydroxysteroid dehydrogenase. This factor was termed interleukin-3 based on its predominant production by mitogen-stimulated T lymphocytes and its presumed role in early T cell differentiation (Ihle and Weinstein, 1986). It was first purified to homogeneity from conditioned media of the murine myelomonocytic cell line WEHI-3B. Subsequent studies demonstrated that IL-3 promotes the proliferation of primitive erythroid (BFU-E), megakaryocyte (CFU-Mk) and granulocyte–macrophage progenitor cells (CFU-GM) and mast cells, activities previously shown for a variety of T-cell-derived factors. Furthermore, murine IL-3 supported proliferation of pluripotential murine cell lines and enhanced the proliferation of spleen colony-forming units (CFU-S) in the mouse, which at that time were considered to be equivalent to the pluripotential haemopoietic stem cell. Based on this broad spectrum of activities, IL-3 has been variously referred to as mast cell growth factor, P-cell-stimulating factor, stem-cell-activating factor and burst-promoting activity (Yang and Clark, 1989). The most commonly used synonym is multi-CSF, referring to the ability of IL-3 to stimulate proliferation of multiple lineages of haemopoietic progenitor cells.

Extensive biological characterization of IL-3 not only in vitro but in animal studies was made possible by the isolation of cDNA clones for murine IL-3 and the subsequent large-scale production of recombinant material. Recombinant murine IL-3 was found to exhibit the same biological activities as the natural, biochemically purified material, and proved to be effective in stimulating haemopoiesis in normal and myelosuppressed animals (Metcalf *et al.*, 1986; Broxmeyer *et al*, 1989).

Human and gibbon IL-3 proteins were found to differ by only 11 amino acids, and were therefore expected to possess similar biological activities; the low homology between IL-3 sequences of other species explains the species specificity of this molecule (Yang *et al.*, 1986; Donahue *et al.*, 1988). The

Table 7.1. *Characteristics of IL-3*

Produced by	Activated T-lymphocytes, keratinocytes, NK-cells, mast cells, monocytes
Target cells	Multipotent progenitor cells; progenitor cells of erythroid, megakaryocytic, eosinophil, granulocyte, macrophage and mast cell lineage; macrophages, eosinophils, basophils, keratinocytes
Gene location	Human chromosome 5q23–33
Protein size	133 amino acids
Molecular weight	14–28 kDa (varies with glycosylation)

human IL-3 gene is located on the long arm of chromosome 5, in close proximity to the genes encoding GM-CSF, M-CSF, the M-CSF receptor, IL-4 and IL-5 and a variety of other growth factor or receptor genes (Yang and Clark, 1989). The significance of this clustering of genes is currently unknown. Structurally mature human IL-3 protein consists of 133 amino acids and has a predicted molecular mass of 14-28 kDa, depending on the degree of glycosylation. While the functions of the carbohydrate chains are not known, the molecule's biological activity in vitro and in vivo is independent of its glycosylation (Table 7.1).

Originally, IL-3 was thought to be produced exclusively by T lymphocytes or T cell tumour lines, quite unlike GM-CSF, which is produced by T cells, endothelial cells, epithelial cells and fibroblasts. Lymphocytes do not produce IL-3 constitutively, but only after prior stimulation. Even in T cells, however, IL-3 gene expression is limited to a small fraction of T cells, and seems to be more stringently regulated than the expression of the other T-cell-derived lymphokines. Interestingly, lymphocytes and NK cells capable of expressing IL-3 mRNA (and, for that matter, GM-CSF mRNA) could be greatly expanded by IL-2, suggesting a possible physiological mechanism for amplifying production of these factors in vivo. Mast cells and, in more recent studies, human thymic epithelial cells and possibly monocytes were also shown to express IL-3 mRNA and produce biologically active IL-3. All studies to date have failed to detect IL-3 mRNA in human bone-marrow-derived stromal cells (Yang and Clark, 1989).

Mechanisms of action of IL-3 and IL-3 receptor

The intracellular mechanisms by which IL-3 induces its biological effects are poorly understood, although there is evidence that signal transduction involves tyrosine phosphorylation of intracellular protein substrates identical to those stimulated by direct activators of protein kinase C. Preceding all signal transduction events is the binding of IL-3 to specific cell surface receptors. High- and low-affinity IL-3 receptors have been identified in different types of human haemopoietic cells. Molecular cloning of various cytokine receptors has established that structurally, the receptors for IL-3, GM-CSF and G-CSF are distantly related to each other and, together with the receptors for IL-2, IL-4, IL-6, IL-7, prolactin and growth hormone, form a newly defined receptor superfamily (Nicola, 1991).

In vitro studies

Identification of the structurally related mammalian homologue of the murine multipotential haemopoietin IL-3 raised the question of a functional relationship between the two species. Analysis of gibbon and human IL-3 on human haemopoietic cells in vitro revealed a broad range of haemopoietic activities resembling that in the murine system. In semisolid media, human and gibbon IL-3 supported formation of colonies derived from human multipotential and committed erythroid, granulocytic, macrophage, eosinophil and megakaryocyte progenitors (Morstyn and Burgess, 1988). Furthermore, IL-3 was found to stimulate even more primitive progenitor cells, detected as CFU-blast, high proliferative potential colony-forming cells (HPP-CFC) or pre-CFU in modified semisolid cultures. In these assays, IL-3 was consistently more effective in stimulating colony formation by pluripotent blast cells than GM-CSF, the multilineage growth factor most closely resembling IL-3 in terms of its haemopoietic activities. This observation suggested that the targets of IL-3 include more primitive progenitors than those of GM-CSF. Remarkably, the stimulatory effect of IL-3 alone on colony formation was diminished or lost in serum-free culture, or when highly purified progenitor cells were used as targets, thereby eliminating accessory cell effects. Interestingly, in the absence of accessory cells, IL-3-induced colony formation could be restored by the addition of a late-acting CSF, e.g. G-CSF, GM-CSF or IL-5. This is analogous to the erythroid system, in which the presence of erythropoietin in addition to IL-3 or GM-CSF is mandatory for the complete development of erythroid cells. Studies demonstrating a declining sensitivity of murine multipotential haemopoietic progenitors during their differentiation and the loss of responsiveness with differentiation

Table 7.2. *Effects of IL-3 on cell functions (reviewed by Valent et al., 1990)*

Monocytes/macrophages	Enhances survival, phagocytosis, ADCC, production of G-CSF, GM-CSF, TNF
Eosinophils	Enhances survival, phagocytosis, ADCC, H_2O_2 production
Basophils	Enhances survival, leukotriene formation, histamine synthesis and release, adhesion to vascular endothelium

ADCC, antibody-dependent cytotoxicity.

in the human myeloid series provided further evidence that IL-3 preferentially stimulates proliferation of more primitive progenitors. Terminal differentiation then requires the additional presence of late-acting growth factors. Interactions of potential clinical relevance between IL-3 and other cytokines have also been observed at the level of more primitive haemopoietic progenitors, where IL-3 acts synergistically with both IL-6 and IL-1 in supporting early blast cell colony formation. Thus, an extensive body of in vitro experimentation indicates that the participation of several sequentially acting haemopoietic factors is required for supporting the complete developmental programme of early haemopoietic progenitors. While there is evidence that IL-3 may affect the direction of differentiation of such early progenitors, it does not appear to be able to induce stem cell renewal in culture.

Receptor binding studies and bioassays have extended the known target cell range of IL-3 to include terminally differentiated eosinophils, basophils, connective tissue-type mast cells, macrophages and keratinocytes (Table 7.2). IL-3 stimulates eosinophil complement-mediated phagocytosis, antibody-dependent cytotoxicity (ADCC) and superoxide anion production. It has been shown to enhance macrophage cytotoxicity and microbicidal and tumouricidal properties; in some cases this requires at least a second activating signal. Cytokine secretion by monocytic cells can also be stimulated by IL-3. IL-3 further augments the growth and survival of human basophils in liquid culture of bone marrow cells, and enhances their production of allergic compounds. Stimulation of bone marrow cells with IL-3 has led to greatly increased intracellular histamine levels, correlating with the number of basophilic granulocytes. Thus, IL-3 is a potential mediator of allergic reactions, although it is not yet known whether it is produced in systemically or locally significant amounts in atopic individuals. Interestingly, macaca species receiving extremely high doses of IL-3 developed urticaria and vasculitic symptoms (Mayer et al., 1989), which resolved with termination of IL-3 administration. Despite histamine release in vivo, no such reactions have been observed in humans treated with IL-3, but need to be considered when designing clinical trials (Merget et al., 1990).

High affinity receptors for IL-3 decline with progressive differentiation within the neutrophilic pathway, and are absent from mature neutrophils, corresponding to the unresponsiveness of this cell type to IL-3. Likewise, mature T and B lymphocytes are unresponsive to IL-3, as are endothelial cells and fibroblasts (Nicola, 1991).

Role of IL-3 in leukaemia

IL-3 stimulates proliferation of blast cells in a subset of human acute myeloid leukaemias (Herrmann and Vellenga, 1990) and, together with other cytokines, such as IL-7, induces clonal proliferation of blasts in a small fraction of pre-B acute lymphoblastic leukaemia. Several leukaemic cell lines responsive to, or dependent on IL-3 have been established. It has also been shown that the blast cells in a number of primary myeloid leukaemias express IL-3 mRNA and produce the IL-3 protein. Because of these data and the known role of colony-stimulating factors in the proliferative regulation of myeloid progenitors, IL-3 as well as the other CSFs were speculated to be of major importance in leukaemogenesis. In a murine model in which mice exhibited profound chronic elevations of IL-3 after being repopulated with haemopoietic cells containing abnormally regulated IL-3 cDNA, massive myeloid hyperplasia with peripheral blood leucocytosis including less mature and mature neutrophils, eosinophils, monocytes and basophils developed. Animals with leucocytosis also developed hepatomegaly and splenomegaly due to infiltration by mature granulocytic cells, but no leukaemic cells evolved during the lifespan of the animals (Lübbert et al., 1990). On the other hand, when dysregulated IL-3 cDNA was inserted into transformed cell lines dependent on IL-3, leukaemic transformation promptly occurred, indicating that with pre-existing abnormalities, the IL-3 gene is capable of acting as a cellular proto-oncogene.

Preclinical studies

Studies in which mice (Kindler et al., 1986; Broxmeyer et al., 1989), rats (Ulich et al., 1989) or primates (Donahue et al., 1988; Geissler et al., 1990;

Wagemaker *et al.*, 1990) received intraperitoneal, intravenous or subcutaneous injections with IL-3 demonstrated that IL-3 generally stimulated cell proliferation in those lineages known from in vitro studies to be responsive to proliferative stimulation by IL-3. IL-3 given intraperitoneally to mice resulted in a 10-fold elevation of peripheral blood eosinophils and a 3-fold elevation of neutrophils and monocytes. The peritoneal cellularity increased, accompanied by the functional activation of peritoneal macrophages. An expansion of the progenitor compartment was located primarily in the spleen, whereas IL-3 administration had little effect on the cellularity and progenitor content in the bone marrow. The mast cell and megakaryocyte content in the spleen increased, as did the number of nucleated erythroid cells and maturing myeloid cells, leading to splenic enlargement. Mature granulocytes and macrophages also accumulated in non-haemopoietic organs such as the lung and liver.

Single doses of IL-3 administered to normal mice resulted, within hours, in increased cycling rates (percentage of cells in S-phase) of CFU-GEMM, BFU-E and CFU-GM and in increased numbers of haemopoietic progenitors in the marrow and spleen. In this regard, IL-3 acted synergistically with other CSFs (Broxmeyer *et al.*, 1989). In sublethally irradiated mice, the administration of IL-3 for a period of 7 days enhanced the number of bone marrow progenitors more than 10-fold above those of untreated controls, to a near normal level. Both erythroid and myeloid lineages were affected to the same extent.

In several studies of normal healthy primates, IL-3 treatment resulted in a somewhat delayed and less pronounced increase in leucocytes as compared to the more lineage-restricted growth factors G-CSF and GM-CSF. Neutrophils, basophils and eosinophils were the predominant cell type contributing to this increase, while platelet and reticulocyte counts were increased to a more variable degree. In a cynomolgus monkey model of chemotherapy-induced myelosuppression, the administration of IL-3 (20 μg/kg/day as continuous i.v. infusion or twice daily subcutaneous bolus injection) for 14 days following treatment with cyclophosphamide or 5-FU, resulted in an amelioration of the degree of leucopenia and an enhanced recovery of the WBC compared with control animals. This was associated with a significant basophilia and eosinophilia, similar to the studies in rhesus monkeys mentioned above. It is therefore of interest that the predominant toxicity of IL-3 was a moderate, self-limiting allergic symptomatology involving localized facial swelling and a pruritic rash (Mayer *et al.*, 1989). Mild splenomegaly developed in some animals. Comparison of studies utilizing continuous intravenous infusion or subcutaneous bolus injections of equivalent doses of IL-3 indicate that these two modes of administration exert essentially the same haematological effects.

In view of the synergistic activity of IL-3 and other growth factors in vitro and in non-primate in vivo models, IL-3 was tested in conjunction with GM-CSF in healthy macaques. While IL-3 alone caused an only modest increase in leucocyte counts, it greatly potentiated the animals' response to subsequent administration of GM-CSF (Mayer *et al.*, 1989). This finding was corroborated by a subsequent study, which also showed that subcutaneous administration of IL-3 to rhesus monkeys greatly increased the levels of circulating progenitor cells, and that this increase was enhanced synergistically by the subsequent administration of GM-CSF (Geissler *et al.*, 1990). IL-3 was not only found to improve the response to GM-CSF with a more pronounced increase of neutrophil counts, but also to erythropoietin with a more rapid increase in haemoglobin levels (Umemura *et al.*, 1989), and to IL-6 with higher increases of platelet numbers (Ulich *et al.*, 1989). These findings support the concept that IL-3 acts on an immature cell population, which can then be stimulated to proliferate and terminally differentiate in response to a second, later-acting factor.

CLINICAL APPLICATIONS OF IL-3

Phase-I trial

In the initial phase-I trial, the treatment schedule consisted of increasing dose levels of IL-3, i.e. 60 $\mu g/m^2$, 125 $\mu g/m^2$, 250 $\mu g/m^2$ and 500 $\mu g/m^2$, administered by subcutaneous bolus injection daily for 15 days (Ganser *et al.*, 1990a; 1991b). Treatment with IL-3 clearly induced a multilineage response with an increase in leucocytes, platelets and reticulocytes (Table 7.3). In response to daily subcutaneous administration of IL-3, the leucocyte counts rose in a dose-dependent but delayed manner, with mean peak leucocyte counts 1.1 times greater than baseline at a daily dose of 60 $\mu g/m^2$ to 2.8 times above baseline at 500 $\mu g/m^2$ at the end of the second week. The increase in leucocytes was primarily due to a rise of segmented neutrophils, eosinophils and lymphocytes, e.g. the neutrophil counts increased by more than $5 \times 10^9/l$ at 500 $\mu g/m^2$. After discontinuation of treatment, neutrophil numbers gradually returned to baseline levels within 1–2 weeks. However, in individual patients they could remain elevated for up to 2 weeks. Reversible eosinophilia occurred at all dose levels ranging from $1 \times 10^9/l$ to $3.75 \times 10^9/l$. Basophil counts also increased but did not reach pathological levels. Both T

Table 7.3. *Clinical trials of interleukin-3*

Clinical condition	No. of patients	Dosage of IL-3 (μg/m^2/day)	Major findings
Advanced malignancy (Ganser *et al.*, 1990a)	19	60–500 × 15	Increased PMN, eos, lympho, baso, plt, reti; increase of serum IgM; increased marrow cellularity; stimulation of CFU-GEMM, BFU-E, CFU-GM
Secondary bone marrow failure (Ganser *et al.*, 1990a)	9	30–500 × 15	Increased PMN, eos, plt, reti, lympho; increase in serum IgM; increase in marrow cellularity
Secondary marrow failure (Kurzrock *et al.*, 1991)	3	125–00 × 23-28	Increased PMN
Myelodysplastic syndromes (Ganser *et al.*, 1990)	9	250–500 × 15	Increased PMN, eos, plt, reti, lympho, serum IgM, IgA; increase in marrow cellularity
Myelodysplastic syndromes (Dunbar *et al.*, 1990)	10	125 × 28	Increased PMN, plt, reti
Myelodysplastic syndromes (Kurzrock *et al.*, 1991)	13	30–1000 × 4-28	Increased PMN, eos, plt, reti
Aplastic anaemia (Ganser *et al.*, 1990c)	9	250–500 × 15	Increased PMN (5 of 9), plt (1 of 9), reti (4 of 9), increased marrow cellularity (3 of 9)
Aplastic anaemia (Kurzrock *et al.*, 1991)	8	30–1000 × 28	Increased PMN (1 of 9), eos (1 of 9), reti (1 of 9), plt (1 of 9)
Diamond-Blackfan anaemia (Dunbar *et al.*, 1991)	6	60–125 × 28	Increased reti (3/5), decreased need for transfusions

Abbreviations: baso, basophils; eos, eosinophils; lympho, lymphocytes; plt, platelets; PMN, polymorphonuclear neutrophils; reti, reticulocytes.

helper and T suppressor lymphocytes were increased between 1.9 and 2.4 times after treatment. Stimulation of the B-lymphocyte lineage was evident from the increase in serum IgM levels, while serum IgG, IgA and IgE did not change significantly. The reason why only the IgM and not the IgG, IgA and IgE gradients increased after IL-3 is unknown, as IL-3 has been shown to induce IgG production by human B lymphocytes in vitro. But the increase of serum levels of IL–6, soluble IL-2 receptor and B2-microglobulin in patients receiving IL–3 is indicative for a broader immunomodulatory action of this cytokine (Lindemann et al., 1991 a,b).

The most important and clinically promising response to IL-3 was the increase in platelet and reticulocyte counts, which could be of value after chemotherapy or bone marrow transplantation. Dose-dependent increases in platelet counts were observed in 15 of 18 evaluable patients, ranging from 1.3-fold at 60 $\mu g/m^2$ to 1.9-fold at 250 $\mu g/m^2$. The time interval until the platelet count actually rose was equally dose-dependent, starting earlier at the higher dosages. The platelet counts sometimes continued to rise for an additional week after discontinuation of IL-3 treatment before returning to base line levels over a period of 2–3 weeks. A stimulation of erythropoiesis with an increase in reticulocyte counts was observed in 14 patients, but the increase in reticulocytes was followed by a rise of the haemoglobin level by more than 1 g/dl in only 2 out of 18 patients.

Bone marrow cellularity increased along with increases in megakaryocytes and eosinophils but not in basophils (Falk et al., 1991). Granulopoiesis was shifted to the left with increased percentages of promyelocytes and myelocytes. The observed decrease in the percentage of lymphoid cells in the bone marrow was only relative and was due to an expansion of myelopoiesis.

Following treatment with IL-3, the percentage of actively cycling bone marrow CFU-GEMM, BFU-E and CFU-GM increased significantly (Ottmann et al., 1990). The relative frequencies of the progenitor cells, however, remained unchanged. Mean levels of circulating CFU-GEMM and CFU-GM were increased after 7 days of treatment but returned to near baseline levels after 15 days of therapy. In contrast, peripheral blood BFU-E was reduced in the majority of patients by the end of the second week.

The clear, but somewhat delayed, increase in the leucocyte, reticulocyte and platelet counts induced by IL-3 is consistent with the concept that IL-3 exerts its principle action at the level of multipotent and committed haemopoietic progenitor cells and not at the level of morphologically recognizable myeloid precursor cells in the bone marrow. This is further supported by the data on the cell cycle status of the progenitor cells CFU-GEMM, BFU-E and CFU-GM. As the increments in mature blood cells were moderate, a combination of IL-3 with later-acting cytokines, e.g. GM-CSF, G-CSF or erythropoietin, might improve the haemopoietic effects of IL-3.

IL-3 in patients with bone marrow failure

Infections and bleeding are the most frequent causes of death in patients with bone marrow failure secondary to chemotherapy/radiotherapy, with myelodysplastic disorders or with aplastic anaemia. In contrast to the rapid rise in leucocyte counts which can be obtained by treatment with GM-CSF or G-CSF (Morstyn and Burgess, 1988), treatment of anaemia and severe thrombocytopenia has been dependent solely on red blood cell and platelet transfusion in patients unresponsive to conventional therapy. Based on the experience with IL-3 in the phase-I trial, IL-3 was administered to patients with multilineage haemopoietic failure, especially to those with severe thrombocytopenia in a subsequent study.

Secondary haemopoietic failure

Bone marrow hypoplasia due to prolonged chemotherapy for cancer or bone marrow infiltration by tumour cells proved to be especially responsive to treatment with IL-3 (Ganser *et al.*, 1990a). In comparison to patients with preserved haemopoietic function treated in the phase I trial, the rise in circulating leucocytes was more delayed, but eventually seven of eight treated and evaluable patients achieved neutrophil counts above 2×10^9/l, and no patient had a count below 0.5×10^9/l after treatment. The median time to peak neutrophil counts was 19 days (range, 6–50). The response to IL-3 was even more remarkable in three patients who had previously been treated with GM-CSF without achieving a durable improvement of haemopoietic function. A stimulation of thrombopoiesis resulting in a 1.3- to 14.3-fold (mean, 6-fold) increase in circulating platelet numbers occurred in five of the eight patients. This increase resulted in discontinuation of platelet transfusions in two out of three patients who had been dependent on repeated substitution. Reticulocyte counts responded to administration of IL-3 in six of eight patients, however, the necessity of red blood cell transfusions was not reduced.

In contrast to treatment with GM-CSF, which had previously been given to some of the patients, IL-3 appears to stimulate and expand the progenitor pools leading to prolonged and even sustained improvement of bone marrow function with increased marrow cellularity and improvement of blood cell formation. Whether IL-3 improves the function of the marrow stromal cells is not known, but could be a feasible explanation for its prolonged effects.

Myelodysplastic syndromes (MDS)

Pronounced responses of the leucocyte counts to IL-3 injections were observed in nine patients with MDS treated in a phase-II trial. Significant increases in total leucocytes, neutrophils, eosinophils, basophils, lymphocytes and monocytes occured after daily dosages of 250 $\mu g/m^2$ or 500 $\mu g/m^2$ (Ganser et al., 1990b; 1991a). Neutrophilic granulocytes increased in all nine patients from a mean of $1.35 \times 10^9/l$ (range, 0.29-2.42) to $2.66 \times 10^9/l$ (range 0.3–9.38) immediately after the end of IL-3 therapy. After discontinuation of IL-3 treatment, leucocyte counts gradually decreased to baseline levels. The response of reticulocytes was diverse. In a single patient a substantial increase of reticulocyte counts was associated with a transient reduction of transfusion requirements. In contrast, two patients with 5q-syndrome had a markedly diminished erythropoiesis following IL-3 treatment, resulting in increased transfusion requirements. Increases in platelet counts, accompanied by a reduced bleeding tendency, were seen in two out of four profoundly thrombocytopenic patients, allowing a short-term discontinuation of platelet transfusions; however, repeated courses of IL-3 in three patients were only partially effective. Transient increases in circulating blast cells occurred in two patients, not exceeding 1% in the differential count. In an additional patient, the increase in circulating blast cells was sustained and paralleled by a rise of blast cells in the bone marrow.

The leucocyte response to IL-3 was comparable to that observed in patients with normal haemopoiesis. The increase in platelet and reticulocyte counts induced by IL-3 was, however, only moderate, probably due to the design of the trial only allowing for short-term treatment courses. Nevertheless, two out of four profoundly thrombocytopenic transfusion-dependent patients had a clinical benefit from a modest increase of platelet counts in that they did not require platelet transfusions for a period of 4 months. IL-3 therefore appears to be at least as efficient as both GM-CSF and G-CSF with regard to its action on thrombopoiesis (Ganser et al., 1990a). The recently reported results of other phase I/II trials seem to support these data further (Dunbar et al., 1990; Kurzrock et al., 1991). Future trials should address the question whether prolonged treatment with IL-3, either alone or in combination with later-acting cytokines, will lead to a more pronounced increase of peripheral cell counts.

Aplastic anaemia

In the initial phase-I/II trial in nine patients, treatment with IL-3 induced a moderate haemopoietic response with an increase in leucocytes in the majority of the treated patients, all but one of whom were transfusion-dependent (Ganser *et al.,* 1990c). Seven out of nine patients had a severe form of the disease, seven patients had already been pretreated with immunosuppressive agents, while two had also received recombinant GM-CSF without any lasting improvements of peripheral blood counts.

The moderate haematological responses to treatment with IL-3 included one patient who showed a transient increase in platelet numbers up to a peak count of $31 \times 10^9/l$ on day 32 resulting in a transient reduction of platelet transfusion requirements. Despite some minor increase of reticulocyte counts, this did not translate into a reduction of transfusion requirements. Neutrophil counts increased at least 2-fold in five of the nine patients. Similar data were obtained by Kurzrock *et al.* (1991).

The responses of the leucocyte counts to IL-3 were comparable to those observed in patients treated with GM-CSF (Nissen *et al.*, 1991), although in patients with less severe forms of the disease mean increases in cell counts were smaller in response to IL-3 than to GM-CSF. However, the responses reported after GM-CSF treatment were observed following several successive cycles, while IL-3 treatment was given for only one course. The increases in leucocyte counts were not sustained after the end of treatment despite marked increases in cellularity and in myelopoiesis in the bone marrow in some patients, probably indicating that IL-3 should be administered continuously for prolonged periods in future trials and in combination with immunosuppressive therapy. Whether prolonged cytokine therapy alone will be able to restore the haemopoietic stem cell pool to normal appears questionable and awaits clinicial confirmation.

IL-3 may produce beneficial clinical effects in patients with Diamond–Blackfan anaemia. In a pilot study of six patients, daily subcutaneous administration of IL-3 at a dosage of 60 or 125 $\mu g/m^2$ led to a reduction of transfusion dependency in several cases previously unresponsive to GM-CSF (Dunbar *et al.,* 1991).

Adverse effects of recombinant human IL-3

Side-effects of IL-3 were mild and included fever in the majority of patients, which was usually more pronounced during the first few days of therapy. Headache accompanied by stiffness of the neck was a common finding at higher dosages. Other more common adverse effects were chills, bone pain and mild local erythema at the site of the subcutaneous application of IL-3. Thrombocytopenia was noted sporadically at high doses.

Facial flushing occurred in a couple of patients, and a prompt release of histamine from the circulating basophils could be readily demonstrated (Merget et al., 1990). The histamine release was nearly complete at 3 h after the first injection of rhIL-3. Normal histamine levels per basophil were only observed again after the end of the 15-day treatment cycle. However, there were no further side-effects attributable to histamine release.

Platelet counts may show a transient reduction at high IL-3 dosages, as shown in two patients with MDS and in one patient with aplastic anaemia treated at the 250 μg/m^2 or 500 μg/m^2 dose levels. The platelet count returned to pretreatment values within 2 weeks of discontinuation of IL-3 application. The reason for the drop in platelet counts at higher dosages is still obscure, but most probably due to increased consumption, as the incidence of megakaryocytes in the bone marrow was regularly increased.

Because IL-3 receptors are also found on malignant haemopoietic and lymphoid cells (Herrmann and Vellenga, 1990), it was not surprising to observe increases in the number of circulating atypical B lymphocytes in one patient with follicular, mixed small cleaved and large cell lymphoma and in one patient with diffuse large cell lymphoma. The latter patient also developed palpable lymph nodes and an increase in spleen size, which were all reversible within 2 weeks of discontinuation of IL-3. The transient increase in circulating lymphoma cells and in the size of the lymph nodes with regression after discontinuation of IL-3 treatment indicates that the lymphoma cells apparently were receptive to IL-3 stimulation. No increase in paraprotein levels was observed in the two patients with multiple myeloma, nor were there any definite growth responses of the malignant tissue in patients with solid tumours, despite the possibility that IL-3 receptors are expressed on non-haemopoietic tumour cells (Berdel et al., 1989). From these initial data, IL-3 should be used with caution in patients with myeloid and lymphoid malignancies, as stimulation of tumour growth is a definite possibility.

Future prospects of IL-3 in clinical practice

Although many questions remain, the initial clinical studies indicate that IL-3 is a potent and well-tolerated stimulus of thrombopoiesis,

Table 7.4. *Potential therapeutic role of IL-3*

1) Treatment of insufficient haemopoiesis, especially thrombopoiesis:
   Acceleration of haematological recovery following chemo/radiotherapy
   Correction of primary bone marrow failure:
   aplastic anaemia
   Diamond–Blackfan anaemia
   myelodysplastic syndromes
2) Improvement of cell harvesting from bone marrow or peripheral
   blood for haemopoietic stem cell transplantation
3) Priming of leukaemic cells for cytostatic drug treatment
4) Priming of haemopoietic progenitor cells for the action of later acting
   cytokines/molecules (GM-CSF, G-CSF, M-CSF, IL-6, EPO, haemin)

leucocytopoiesis and erythropoiesis in man, acting predominantly on the early haemopoietic progenitor cells. It may be useful in the treatment of chemotherapy/radiotherapy-induced or disease-related pancytopenic disorders, either alone or in combination with later acting haemopoietic growth factors by decreasing transfusion requirements and reducing the risk of infections (Table 7.4). It might therefore be used following regular chemotherapy or radiotherapy with known myelosuppressive activity or after bone marrow transplantation. As IL-3 is known to recruit haemopoietic progenitors to become more responsive to lineage-restricted cytokines (Lübbert *et al.*, 1990), combinations with either GM-CSF or G-CSF could lead to an accelerated regeneration of granulocytes, and combinations with erythropoietin or interleukin-6 to an accelerated production of red blood cells and platelets, respectively.

Although IL-3 alone is not able to expand the circulating progenitor cell pool when given to patients with normal haemopoiesis (Ottmann *et al.*, 1990), the situation might be different if it is given in the regenerative period after regular chemotherapy. Preclinical and initial clinical findings, however, indicate that the combination of IL-3 and other cytokines, e.g. GM-CSF, is an especially effective way to increase the number of circulating haemopoietic progenitor cells CFU-GEMM, BFU-E and CFU-GM, which can then be harvested by leucapheresis for autologous stem cell transfusions (Brugger *et al.*, 1992; Ganser *et al.*, 1992).

The potential clinical use of IL-3 is not restricted to the mitigation of therapy-induced cytopenic states but can be extended to patients with myelodysplastic syndromes in whom IL-3 can reverse thrombocytopenia at least in a subgroup of patients, and in patients with cytopenia associated with viral infection. In patients with severe aplastic anaemia, IL-3 alone appears to be quite ineffective, but combinations with immunosuppressive therapy or other haemopoietic cytokines have to be tested; in contrast, it appears to be active in the rather rare congenital Diamond–Blackfan anaemia.

As leukaemic blast cells are frequently dependent on either IL-3, GM-CSF, G-CSF, or a combination of these factors, it is conceivable to interfere in pre- and post-receptor events for therapeutic effect. This could be done by the development of mutated forms of the growth factors with antagonistic properties that would suppress leukaemic cell proliferation. A different approach for the use of IL-3 was derived from in vitro studies where IL-3 can be used to induce leukaemic cells into active cell cycle and to render them more sensitive to the action of cell-cycle-specific drugs.

Finally, the development of IL-3 or IL-3 receptor antagonists might be helpful in the therapy or prevention of graft-versus-host disease and allergic disorders, i.e. clinical conditions at least partly mediated through the action of IL-3.

REFERENCES

Berdel WE, Danhauser-Riedl S, Steinhauser G and Winton EF (1989). Various human hematopoietic growth factors (Interleukin-3, GM-CSF, G-CSF) stimulate clonal growth of non hematopoietic tumor cells. *Blood.* **73**, 80–3.

Broxmeyer HE, Williams DE, Cooper S *et al.* (1989). Comparative effects in vivo of recombinant murine interleukin 3, natural murine colony-stimulating factor-1, and recombinant murine granulocyte-macrophage colony-stimulating factor on myelopoiesis in mice. *J Clin Invest.* **79**, 721–30.

Brugger W, Bross K, Frisch J et al. (1992). Mobilization of peripheral blood progenitor cells by sequential administration of interleukin-3 and granulocyte-macrophage colony-stimulating factor following polychemotherapy with etoposide, ifosfamide, and cisplatin. *Blood.* **79**, 1193–200

Donahue RE, Seehra J, Metzger M *et al.* (1988). Human IL-3 and GM-CSF act synergistically in stimulating hematopoiesis in primates. *Science.* **241**, 1820–3.

Dunbar CE, Smith D, Kimball J *et al.* (1990). Sequential treatment with recombinant human growth factors to compare activity of GM-CSF and IL3 in the treatment of primary myelodysplasia. *Blood.* **76 (Suppl 1)**, 141a-46a.

Dunbar CE, Smith DA, Kimball J *et al.* (1991). Treatment of Diamond-Blackfan anaemia with haematopoietic growth factors, granulocyte-macrophage colony stimulating factor and interleukin-3: sustained remissions following IL-3. *Br J Haematol.* **79**, 316–21

Falk S, Seipelt G, Ganser A *et al.* (1991). Bone marrow findings after treatment with recombinant human interleukin-3. *Am J Clin Pathol.* **95**, 355–62.

Ganser A, Lindemann A, Seipelt G *et al.* (1990a). Effect of recombinant human interleukin-3 in patients with normal hematopoiesis and in patients with bone marrow failure. *Blood* **76**, 666–76.

Ganser A, Seipelt G, Lindemann A *et al.* (1990b). Effects of recombinant human interleukin-3 in patients with myelodysplastic syndromes. *Blood.* **76**, 455–62.

Ganser A, Lindemann A, Seipelt G *et al.* (1990c) Effects of recombinant human interleukin-3 in aplastic anemia. *Blood.* **76**, 1287–1292.

Ganser A, Seipelt G and Hoelzer D (1991a). The role of GM-CSF, interleukin-3 and erythropoietin in myelodysplastic syndromes. *Am J Clin Oncol (CCT).* **14 (Suppl 1)**, 34–9.

Ganser A, Lindemann A, Seipelt G *et al.* (1991b). Clinical effects of recombinant humen interleukin-3. *Am J Clin Onc (CCT).* **14 (Suppl 1)**, 51–63.

Ganser A, Lindemann A, Ottmann OG *et al.* (1992). Sequential in vivo treatment with two recombinant human hematopoietic growth factors (interleukin-3 and granulocyte-macrophage colony-stimulating factor) as a new therapeutic modality to stimulate hematopoiesis: Results of a phase I study. *Blood.* **79**, in press

Garnick MB and O'Reilly RJ (1989). Clinical promise of new hematopoietic growth factors: M-CSF, IL-3, IL-6. *Hematol/Oncol Clin North Am.* **3**, 495–509.

Geissler K, Valent P, Mayer P *et al.* (1990). Interleukin-3 expands the circulating pool of haemopoietic stem cells in primates. Synergism with granulocyte macrophage colony stimulating factor. *Blood.* **75**, 2305–11.

Herrmann F and Vellenga E (1990). The role of colony-stimulating factors in acute leukemia. *J Cancer Res Clin Oncol.* **116**, 275–82.

Ihle JN and Weinstein Y (1986). Immunological regulation of hematopoietic/lymphoid stem cell differentiation by interleukin 3. *Adv Immunol.* **39**, 1–50.

Kindler V, Thorens B, de Kossodo S *et al.* (1986). Stimulation of hematopoiesis in vivo by recombinant bacterial murine interleukin 3. *Proc Natl Acad Sci USA.* **83**, 1001–5.

Kurzrock R, Talpaz M, Estrov Z, Rosenblum MG and Gutterman JU (1991). Phase I study of recombinant human interleukin-3 in patients with bone marrow failure. *J Clin Oncol.* **79**, 1241–50.

Lindemann A, Ganser A, Hoelzer D, Mertelsmann A, Herrmann F. (1991a) In vivo administration of recombinant human interleukin 33 elicits an acute phase response involving endogenous synthesis of interleukin-6. *Eur Cytokine Net.* **2**, 1973–6

Lindemann A, Ganser A, Herrmann F *et al.* (1991b) Biologic effects of human interleukin-3 in vivo. *J Clin Oncol.* **9**, 2120–7

Lübbert M, Jonas D and Herrmann F (1990). Animal models for the biological effects of continuous high cytokine levels. *Blut.* **61**, 253–7.

Mayer P, Valent P, Schmidt G *et al.* (1989). The in vivo effect of recombinant human interleukin-3: demonstration of basophil differentiation factor, histamine-producing activity and priming of GM-CSF-responsive progenitors in nonhuman primates. *Blood* . **74**, 613–21.

Merget RD, Maurer AB, Koch U *et al.* (1990). Histamine release from basophils after in vivo application of recombinant human interleukin-3 in man. *Int Arch All Appl Immunol.* **92**, 366–74.

Metcalf D, Begley CG, Johnson GR (1986). Haemopoietic effects of purified bacterially synthesized multi-CSF in normal and marrow-transplanted mice. *Immunobiol.* **172**, 158–67.

Morstyn G and Burgess AW (1988). Haemopoietic growth factors: a review. *Cancer Res.* **48**, 5624–37.

Nicola NA (1991). Receptors for colony-stimulating factors. *Br J Haematol.* **77**, 133–8.

Nissen C, Gratwohl A and Speck B (1991). Management of aplastic anemia. *Eur J Haematol.* **46**, 193–7.

Ottmann OG, Ganser A, Seipelt G *et al.* (1990). Effects of recombinant human interleukin-3 on human hematopoietic progenitor and precursor cells in vivo. *Blood.* **76**, 1494–502.

Ulich TR, del Castillo J, Busser K, Guo K and Yin S (1989). Acute in vivo effects of IL-3 alone and in combination with IL-6 on the blood cells of the circulation and bone marrow. *Am J Pathol.* **135**, 663–70.

Umemura T, al-Khatti A, Donahue RE *et al.* (1989). Effects of interleukin-3 and erythropoietin on in vivo erythropoiesis and F-cell formation in primates. *Blood.* **74**, 1571–6.

Valent P, Geissler K, Sillaber C *et al.* (1990). Why clinicians should be interested in interleukin-3. *Blut.* **61**, 338–45.

Wagemaker G, van Gils FCJM, Burger H *et al.* (1990). Highly increased production of bone marrow derived blood cells by administration of homologous interleukin-3 to rhesus monkeys. *Blood.* **76**, 2235–41.

Yang YC, Ciarletta AB, Temple PA *et al.* (1986). Human IL3 (Multi-CSF): Identification by expression cloning of a novel hematopoietic growth factor related to murine IL-3. *Cell.* **47**, 3–10.

Yang YC and Clark D (1989). Interleukin-3: molecular biology and biologic activities. *Hematol/Oncol Clin North Am.* **3**, 441–52.

8

INTERFERON-ALPHA

D. W. GALVANI and J. C. CAWLEY

INTRODUCTION

Some of the historical aspects of interferon-alpha (IFNα) research have been covered in Professor Cantell's Introduction to this book. In the present chapter we will deal first with the molecular biology and cell biology of IFNα; then we will critically evaluate the clinical applications of this cytokine and discuss the possible mechanisms of action in these areas.

Definition of an interferon An interferon is a protein that exerts virus non-specific, antiviral activity, at least in homologous cells, through cellular metabolic processes involving synthesis of RNA and protein (Anonymous, 1980). To put it another way, when interferon activity is induced within a cell, it protects that cell/organism against further attack from different types of virus; such protection is mediated by interferon-induced proteins that alter viral RNA and protein. This emphasizes a *direct* effect within an affected cell(s). Perhaps it is not surprising, therefore, that such powerful regulatory mechanisms may also alter cell metabolism in certain circumstances, e.g. neoplastic growth. Interferons can have *indirect* effects on cells, when cells of the immune system are stimulated within the vicinity of the cytokine; this is beneficial in terms of control of viral growth, and has a putative role in immunosurveillance for tumour cells. The direct and indirect effects of IFNα do not occur in isolation, but comprise part of a complex cytokine network, as outlined in Chapter 11.

Three broad groups of interferon have been described – IFNα, β and γ (Table 8.1). IFNα has received the most scientific and therapeutic study. Although there are at least 24 subtypes of IFNα, they all share the same receptor and differ only slightly in their individual properties (Greasey *et al.*,

D. W. GALVANI & J. C. CAWLEY

Table 8.1. *Molecular properties of the interferons*

Characteristic	IFNα	IFNβ	IFNγ
Synonym	Leucocyte	Fibroblast	Immune
Subtypes	Over 24	None	None
Source	Leucocytes	Fibroblasts	T lymphocytes
Gene	Ch 9	Ch 9	Ch 12
Homology	30% with β	30% with α	10% with α and β
Molecular weight	16–27 kDa	20 kDa	15–25 kDa
Glycosylation	+	++	+++
Acid stability	+	+	–
Cell surface receptor	Type I	Type I	Type II
Main inducing stimuli	Virus	Virus	Antigen/Mitogen

1988). IFNβ shares the same receptor as IFNα and has a single subtype –what was termed IFNβ–2 has been renamed IL6. IFNβ is very similar to IFNα in its properties, but limited clinical trials have not demonstrated any advantages over IFNα. IFNγ is quite distinct and is a more potent immunomodulator – this is dealt with in Chapter 9.

Interferon assays The biological effect of an IFN is best demonstrated by inhibition of plaque formation within a virus-infected cell monolayer. When compared to a known standard, units of antiviral activity can be ascribed to a sample. Alternatively, radioimmunometric analysis can quantitate specific IFN antigen within a sample. Both measurements are valid and allow calculation of specific activity in units of antiviral activity per mg protein.

MOLECULAR BIOLOGY OF IFNα

The IFNα receptor This high affinity surface receptor has been cloned, and is a glycoprotein of approximately 130 kDa (Grossenberg *et al.*, 1989). Low concentrations of IFNα can initiate an effect, even at low receptor occupancy. After ligand-binding, the receptor complex is internalized, and the ligand is delivered through nuclear pores into the dense chromatin (Grossenberg *et al.*, 1989); the receptor is returned to the cell surface. Receptor biosynthesis occurs continuously at high concentrations of ligand, and can lead to down-regulation of the receptor.

The IFNα receptor is widely distributed on many cell types (Rubinstein and Orchansky, 1986), being particularly abundant on 'hairy cells' found in hairy-cell leukaemia (HCL). This observation may be relevant to the high sensitivity of this leukaemia to IFNα therapy, although receptor kinetics appear similar in both IFNα-sensitive and resistant cells (Morgensen *et al.*, 1989).

Signal transduction Neither cyclic AMP nor prostaglandin breakdown follow IFNα receptor activation (Tovey *et al.*, 1982; Ebsworth *et al.*, 1984). Recent work has shown that activation of the IFNα receptor results in diacylglycerol formation (but not hydrolysis of inositol phospholipids), with translocation of the beta-isoform of protein kinase C (PKC) from cytosol to membrane (Pfeffer *et al.*, 1990). This is in keeping with the work of Yap *et al.* (1986), but the conclusion that PKC is involved in signal transduction has been disputed (Mehmet *et al.*, 1987).

Gene regulation Following viral stimulation, 'IFN regulatory factors' (IRFs) are produced within the cell that bind to the regulatory elements of the IFNα gene. When IFNα itself enters a cell, it produces IRFs that bind to a similar consensus sequence (AGTTTCNNCTCC) both in the IFNα gene and in the genes of IFNα-inducible proteins (Harada *et al.*, 1989). These IRFs can be inhibitory or stimulatory. Thus, IFNα can stimulate transcription of the genes encoding for 2'5' oligonucleotide (2'5'A) synthetase and HLA Class I (Fellous *et al.*, 1982) but inhibits c-*myc* gene transcription (Einat *et al.*, 1985). Effects of IFNα on RNA translation have also been described (Knight *et al.*, 1985).

Cell proteins Several IFNα-induced proteins have been described (Celis, 1987), but only a few have known functional effects. Perhaps the best studied is the induction of 2'5'A synthetase. This enzyme catalyses the production of 2'5'-linked oligomers of adenosine from ATP. These in turn activate a cellular endonuclease which degrades mRNA and rRNA, halting protein synthesis (Williams and Fish, 1985). This has obvious relevance to antiviral activity but may also regulate cellular processes (Kimchi, 1981). Other groups have shown that IFNα stimulates protein kinase A activation, this phosphorylates eukaryotic initiation factor, which inhibits viral replication (Samuel *et al.*, 1984).

Ornithine decarboxylase (ODC) is also activated following IFNα, resulting in reduced polyamine production, which is the rate limiting step in cell growth during the G1 phase of the cell cycle (Sreevalsan, 1980). At the same time mRNA for tubulin appears and this also stabilizes the cell in G1 phase (Fellous *et al.*, 1982). However, it is obvious from cell line work that such mechanisms are only part of a complex set of cell effects, which may be specific for different cell types (Silverman, 1982).

CELL BIOLOGY OF IFNα

Antiviral activity Although 2'5'A-stimulated endonuclease degradation of RNA is a potent antiviral effect, not all viruses are particularly sensitive to this effect (Chebath *et al.,* 1987). IFNα also inhibits viral attachment, penetration, uncoating and budding by producing a variety of metabolic changes within a virus (Williams and Fish, 1985). In mice, IFNα stimulates the Mx protein, which confers increased resistance to viral infection; although this model has been extensively investigated, relevance to human systems is unclear (Staeheli and Haller, 1987).

Cell proliferation The antiproliferative effects of IFN have been studied in most types of normal and tumour-derived human cells (Taylor-Papidimitriou and Rozengurt, 1985). For example, the Daudi lymphoblastoid cell line is arrested in G1 phase, and this is associated with decreased *c-myc* expression (Einat *et al.*, 1985) and with a down-regulation of transferrin receptors (Tamm *et al.,* 1987); the cell is then 'incompetent' to enter further cell cycling (even following removal of IFNα). This has relevance to normal haemopoiesis where autocrine IFNα has been shown to regulate cell growth in mice (Resnitsky *et al.,* 1986). Resistance to IFNα in Daudi-derived cells is independent of IFNα receptor status or inducibility of 2'5'A, but is associated with an absence of suppression of c-*myc* or down-regulation of the transferrin receptor.

In addition to the effects of IFNα on ODC and tubulin mentioned above, other groups have shown that IFNα inhibits DNA polymerization in several types of cell (Tanaka *et al.,* 1987). Such antiproliferative effects observed in vitro, 'may actually have a function in vivo in bringing to an end the proliferative phases that precede a differentiated state' (Morgensen *et al.*, 1989).

Cell differentiation Several differentiation systems have been examined (Rossi, 1985). IFNα inhibits myeloid proliferation and differentiation at high doses, but stimulates cell differentiation at lower concentrations; these effects may be mediated by inhibition of c-*myc* (Resnitsky *et al.*, 1986). The conversion of fibroblasts to adipocytes, and myogenic differentiation may also be inhibited. The mechanism(s) mediating the effects of IFNα on differentiation are not well defined, but it has been suggested that induction of 2'5'A may be involved.

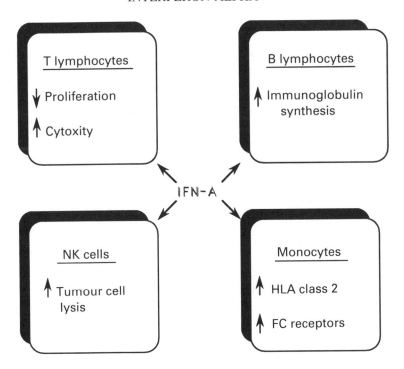

Fig. 8.1. Immune effects of IFNα.

Effects on the immune system Figure 8.1 summarizes the influences of IFNα on immune cells. Although IFNα has an overall suppressive effect on cell division, it strongly stimulates cytotoxic T and natural killer (NK) cell killing in vitro (Griffiths *et al.*, 1989). Such observations have led to the suggestion that enhancement of killer cell activity may account for the antitumour effects of IFNα. However, following clinical administration of IFNα, cytotoxicity is not consistently enhanced when tested ex vivo. Further, IFNα can paradoxically reduce sensitivity of tumour cells to NK lysis (Griffiths *et al.*, 1989a) – clearly IFNα must have other antitumour actions.

Although IFNα inhibits monocyte maturation, it enhances monocyte toxicity by increasing Fc and complement receptors (compare with IFNγ). IFNα has little effect upon neutrophil function, although these cells can produce the cytokine following appropriate stimulation.

IFNα has little effect on B cell proliferation, and this is in keeping with the observation that resting B cells have few IFNα receptors (Dadmarz *et al.*, 1987). At low concentrations of IFNα, immunoglobulin production is enhanced, but the opposite effect may be seen at higher doses.

Table 8.2. *Therapeutically available forms of IFNα*

Trade name	Type of IFNα	Licensed indications
Intron	rh IFNα–2b	HCL, CGL, KS (AIDS-related), condylomata, Hep B
Roferon	rh IFNα–2a	HCL, KS (AIDS-related), CGL, recurrent RCC, Hep B
Wellferon	Lymphoblastoid	HCL, Hep B

Abbreviations: CGL, chronic granulocytic leukaemia; HCL, hairy-cell leukaemia; Hep B, chronic hepatitis B; KS, Kaposis sarcoma; RCC, renal cell carcinoma; rhIFN, recombinant human interferon.

PHARMACOLOGY OF IFNα

Three main preparations of IFNα are generally available in the UK (Table 8.2). All three formulations seem to have similar efficacy, although Wellferon, being a natural cell product, is a mixture of subtypes of IFNα, and may be less immunogenic than the recombinant formulations (Galton et al., 1989). Subcutaneous or intramuscular administration has been preferred to the intravenous route for some time. At doses of 3-5 MU/m², peak serum levels of up to 100 IU/ml can be measured between 3 and 12 h after injection, thus administration in the early evening results in highest levels coinciding with sleep. Steady state levels of up to 90 IU/ml have been detected.The elimination half-life of the agent is a matter of hours, and the kidney is the main site of catabolism and excretion. Interactions with H_2 antagonists, theophyllines and warfarin have been described.

Hypersensitivity to IFNα is an absolute contraindication to further use. However, the agent must be used with caution in patients with known cardiac disease, epilepsy, renal and hepatic decompensation or a history of mental disturbance. Animal studies suggest that IFNα has little teratogenic potential, however, contraception is advised for patients of both sexes receiving the agent. IFNα should only be used in pregnancy if the benefit to the mother is deemed to outweigh the hazard to the fetus.

Children seem more tolerant of doses employed in adults, but the elderly suffer more frequent morbidity. Side-effects are dose-related. Fatigue and flu-like symptoms are the most common complaints at all ages (90%), they can be minimized by administering paracetamol 30 min prior to injection. Nausea and anorexia are seen in two-thirds of patients, and weight should be monitored regularly. Most of these side-effects improve following a few weeks of IFNα therapy and, if troublesome, a reduction or temporary cessation of therapy will improve symptoms. A degree of hair loss is observed in up to 20% of patients and this may persist even after cessation of therapy. Psychological changes during therapy have been well documented and should be reviewed regularly in case dose reduction is required (McDonald, 1987). Psychomotor retardation occurs very rarely in the elderly. Other late side effects have been described, e.g. hypothyroidism, Raynaud's, neuropathy, etc. In patients receiving IFNα for non-haemic conditions, neutropenia and thrombocytopenia may be seen. This frequently stabilizes during continued therapy, but a reduction in dose schedule may be required.

Wellferon is associated with a low incidence of neutralizing antibodies (2%; Galton et al., 1989). Up to one-quarter of patients receiving recombinant products have been associated with the emergence of neutralizing and binding IFN antibodies, higher titres of which can lead to loss of clinical effect and improvement in side-effects (von Wussow et al., 1991a,b). Dose-escalation of the recombinant agent may not overcome this situation, but substitution of the non-recombinant product has been associated with a return to disease responsiveness.

IFNα IN CLINICAL HAEMATO-ONCOLOGY

IFNα in hairy-cell leukaemia

Clinical effects of IFNα After prolonged administration of IFNα, the peripheral cytopenias of this disease are improved in > 80% of patients, whether or not the patient has had a splenectomy (Worman et al., 1985). In particular, the neutropenia of HCL is consistently improved and the incidence of serious infection, formally a major cause of death in the disease, is reduced. Hairy-cell variants are generally unresponsive.

The effects of IFNα on the marrow are less striking and HCs are reduced < 5% in a minority of cases (probably < 10%); even when the HC infiltrate is reduced, considerable fibrosis persists. These beneficial results are achieved with minimal side-effects at 3 MU 3–7 times a week. Occasionally, neutropenia may significantly worsen early in therapy, but this can now be overcome with granulocyte colony-stimulating factor (G-CSF) (Glaspy et al., 1988). Very low dose schedules are ineffective.

Disease activity slowly returns after cessation of therapy, but will normally respond to reintroduction of IFNα therapy. The optimal duration of therapy is not clear but, as significant improvement in marrow function can occur after 6 to 12 months, treatment should probably be continued for at least 1 year.

The different forms of IFNα are probably equally efficacious initially. However, resistance to IFNα-2 in association with neutralizing antibodies has recently been reported in up to one-sixth of HCL patients (von Wussow *et al.*, 1991a). The introduction of non-recombinant IFNα was then associated with a renewed response.

IFNα versus other treatment modalities Deoxycoformycin (dCF) is highly active in HCL (whether or not the patient has had a splenectomy or received IFNα) and produces response rates at least as high as IFNα (Kraut *et al.*, 1986). Furthermore, when dCF is effective, HCs are frequently eradicated from the marrow and, on stopping treatment, the disease does not relapse over substantial periods of follow-up. These impressive results are achieved with relatively small amounts of drug (approximately 12 injections of 4 mg/m^2 over 6 months) and with minimal toxicity.

dCF, therefore, seems to offer a number of advantages over IFNα and should probably be the treatment of choice in the disease. However, dCF is not directly available in the UK, and can only be obtained from the National Cancer Institute (USA) for patients resistant to IFNα or as part of an approved clinical trial.

Very recently, impressive clinical responses have been obtained with chloroxyadenosine (Piro *et al.*, 1990), an agent related to dCF. However, experience with the drug is still limited, and the supply is restricted to the Scripps Clinic in La Jolla, California.

Before the recognition that IFNα and dCF are so effective in HCL, splenectomy was the treatment of first choice. If the spleen is substantially enlarged and if marrow impairment as manifested by marked anaemia is not great, improvement in peripheral cytopenias can be expected following splenectomy. What then is the current place of splenectomy and what is the best overall approach to treatment?

Given that dCF is available in the UK only for patients resistant to IFNα and given that the latter treatment should be prolonged, it seems reasonable to recommend splenectomy, provided that the spleen is substantially enlarged. When the disease eventually recurs, or if there is no response to splenectomy, IFNα therapy should be given. If the spleen is not enlarged, then IFNα should be given from the start. If the disease becomes resistant to IFNα or if the patient becomes intolerant of the agent, dCF (obtained from the NCI) should be given.

Finally, of course, it should be remembered that a small proportion of patients (up to 15%) are asymptomatic and have no peripheral cytopenias – these patients should not be treated.

Mechanism of action of IFNα in HCL HCs are resistant to the cytolytic effects of NK and LAK cells and there is no evidence of generation of CTLs in patients on IFNα (Griffiths and Cawley, 1987, 1988). It therefore seems unlikely that the beneficial effects of the agent are mediated via its immunomodulatory effects on cytotoxic cells.

Although HCs are not killed by exposure to IFNα, they have substantial numbers of IFNα receptors (Dadmarz *et al.*, 1987) and the cytokine inhibits HC proliferation in response to a number of growth stimuli such as BCGF (Griffiths and Cawley, 1989). It therefore seems likely that IFNα acts via its antiproliferative effect on HCs. However, the proliferative stimuli to HCs in vivo are largely unknown and it remains unclear why HCs, among all neoplastic B cells, are so sensitive to the antiproliferative effects of IFNα.

Recent work in this laboratory has shown that direct contact with macrophages and endothelial cells stimulates HC proliferation and that this proliferation is inhibited by IFNα but not IFNγ (Griffiths and Cawley, 1991). It is tempting to speculate that the long-recognized histological association between marrow macrophages and HCs and between endothelial cells and HCs are relevant to the in vivo proliferation of HCs and that this growth stimulus is specifically inhibited by IFNα.

It is difficult to assess the clinical significance of the demonstration that tumour necrosis factor (TNF) is an autocrine growth factor for HCs and that its production is inhibited by IFNα (Cordingley *et al.*, 1989), as identical effects are observed in CLL – a disease which is far less responsive to IFNα. Reports that successful induction of 2'5'A synthetase may correlate with clinical responsiveness to IFNα require further confirmation (De Mel *et al.*, 1990).

IFNα in chronic granulocytic leukaemia

Clinical trials of IFNα IFNα may be effective for initial cytoreduction in chronic granulocytic anaemia (CGL), but it is not consistently so. It is probably better, therefore, to achieve initial control of the disease with hydroxyurea (Hu) or busulphan (Bu) as recommended in the current MRC trial. IFNα can then maintain the white cell count (WCC) between 2 and 5 × 10^9/l in 80% of patients, usually at doses of 3 MU 3 – 7 times per week.

Intermittent Hu or Bu may be employed when the WCC rises above $30 \times 10^9/l$.

The major difference between IFNα and conventional chemotherapy is that the cytokine reduces the Philadelphia positive (Ph+) clone in a significant proportion of patients (Allan and Shepherd, 1987). Thus, Talpaz et al. (1987b) showed that half the patients who responded to IFNα had a reduction in Ph+ marrow metaphases, 10–20% achieving complete karyotypic remission. Other groups are in broad agreement with this, but complete disappearance of the Ph+ clone has been less common (Alimena et al., 1988; Freund et al., 1989). This may reflect patient selection or IFNα scheduling. It appears that the best karyotypic results are obtained by administering IFNα at the highest dose that the patient will reasonably tolerate and by maintaining WCC between 2 and $5 \times 10^9/l$. Major karyotypic responses are generally seen within 12 months of commencing IFNα. Easing the schedule may suboptimize karyotypic response, but may be necessary for patient compliance. The most recent data from the MRC trial of IFNα in CGL show that up to 20% have karyotypic improvement (PR four times as common as CR).

Patients with 'less aggressive' disease seem more responsive to IFNα. Conversely, resistance to IFNα therapy may indicate a poor prognostic group. On this basis it has been suggested that IFNα-responsive patients may have a less pressing requirement for marrow transplantation. When the latter modality is not possible, IFNα may be continued at the maximal tolerated dose with concurrent oral agents if IFNα alone cannot keep the WCC below $5 \times 10^9/l$. Alternatively, to maximize the karyotypic response, the Poitiers group have combined IFNα with low-dose cytosine – these results will prove interesting.

The prospect of a karyotypic normal marrow in CGL raises the possibility of autologous BMT following IFNα therapy. However, because marrow progenitor growth is so poor following IFNα therapy, engraftment may be a problem. Harvesting following a period off IFNα therapy may overcome this, and these possibilities are being explored by the Houston group. It must be added, however, that the same group have demonstrated that when complete karyotypic ablation of the Ph+ clone occurs during IFNα therapy, the polymerase chain reaction can still detect the BCR gene rearrangement in 90% of cases (Goldman, personal communication). Whether this will influence prospects for autologous transplantation remains to be seen.

Initial response rates are similar for each of the formulations of IFNα. Recombinant IFNα may stimulate neutralizing antibodies with associated loss of responsiveness, even at higher doses of the agent. Changing to a non-recombinant formulation has been associated with return of disease responsiveness (von Wussow *et al.*, 1991b).

It is clear that even patients who sustain a fall in their Ph+ clone can still develop acute transformation; there is some evidence that this is more likely to be lymphoid (Talpaz *et al.*, 1987b). However, some patients with a complete karyotypic response can maintain this status off IFNα therapy. It is too early to say if IFNα therapy will improve survival in CGL, and the cytokine needs to be carefully compared with standard therapies. Responses to IFNα will be optimal if the agent is started early in the disease and the highest tolerated maintenance dose is used.

CGL is less responsive to IFNγ than IFNα (Kurzrock *et al.*, 1987). Occasional patients will respond to IFNγ and not IFNα. Thus, combination and cross-over trials are underway to optimize response. There is little place for IFNα in the accelerating phase of CGL.

Mechanism of action Immune mechanisms such as NK cytotoxicity are defective in CGL (Fujiyama and Pattengale, 1985). IFNα therapy does not improve this defect, and clinical responses do not correlate with effects on NK activity (Galvani *et al.*, 1988b). Furthermore, NK cells do not lyse normal or CGL myeloid cells. This is in contrast to LAK cells, which do influence CGL clonal growth (McKinnon *et al.*, 1990), but evidence suggests that IFNα does not influence LAK generation (Griffiths and Cawley, 1988).

IFNα produces a direct inhibition of normal and CGL colony formation (CFU-GM) which is independent of accessory cells (Broxmeyer *et al.*, 1983; Galvani and Cawley, 1989). It appears that, in terms of colony growth and thymidine incorporation, normal and Ph+ clonal growth are equally sensitive to the effects of IFNα. It is possible that currently available assays cannot pick up the differential sensitivity to IFNα that allows Ph– growth to occur at the expense of Ph+ growth. It has been observed in this laboratory that the mature myeloid progenitors are more sensitive to IFNα than the less mature progenitors (Galvani and Cawley, 1989). More mature progenitors are generally more responsive to growth factors. This may be relevant to the mechanism of action of IFNα as it is the mature progenitors that are greatly expanded in CGL (Strife and Clarkson, 1988).

IFNα receptor expression does not correlate with clinical responsiveness to IFNα in CGL (Rosenblum *et al.*, 1986). Similarly, resultant induction of 2'5'A synthetase activity does not correlate with disease response (Schtalrid *et al.*, 1989). IFNα therapy is associated with a reduction of mRNA for the 210 kDa tyrosine kinase of CGL, but whether this reduction is a result of a reduction in the Ph+ clone or of true pathogenic significance is not clear. Secondary cytokine release may also be important, as IFNα stimulates TNF release from macrophages (Pelus et al., 1988). TNF has been described as a regulator of myelopoiesis, and loss of this control may result in blastic transformation in CGL (Duncombe et al., 1989). Therapeutic IFNα may enhance this TNF effect, potentially delaying acceleration and favouring Ph– growth.

Recent work has shown that IFNα can have a marked effect on stromal cells in long-term bone marrow culture (Galvani and Cawley, 1990). It has been suggested that IFNα exposure may alter adhesive properties within the stroma and improve adherence of relatively non-adherent CGL progenitors, thus bringing them back under the influence of normal regulatory mechanisms (Dowding et al., 1991).

Disorders in which IFNα may have a role

Myeloma It appears that IFNα is not superior to standard therapy for primary treatment in myeloma (Ludwig et al., 1986). However, in vitro evidence suggests that IFNα may sensitize myeloma cells to chemotherapeutic agents (Constanzi et al., 1985). Recent clinical work has confirmed that IFNα may be a useful adjunct to chemotherapy, extending response duration, although cardiotoxicity has been observed (Oken et al., 1988).

Most interest now relates to the role of maintenance IFNα in plateau phase. Mandelli et al. (1990) have shown that 3 MU three times a week can halve the relapse rate and double the time to relapse. There is also a suggestion that patients receiving IFNα may respond better to therapy in relapse. The most recent British MRC myeloma trial seeks to confirm these findings.

In relapsed or resistant disease, IFNα alone produces an inconsistent response, often requiring increasing doses, in up to one-third of individuals (Oken et al., 1990). Some patients achieve symptomatic and biochemical improvement but the majority show little benefit. Whether IFNα can act as an adjuvant to chemotherapy in relapsed myeloma remains to be proved.

Lymphoma About half of patients with untreated low grade NHL have a reduction in lymphadenopathy in response to 3 MU IFNα three times a week, and there is a degree of dose responsiveness (Steis et al., 1987). However it is not clear whether IFNα confers any advantage over conventional therapy (O'Connell et al., 1987). Studies are already examining the adjunctive effects of IFNα on conventional therapy and, as in myeloma, there is a suggestion that IFNα may prolong responsiveness (Rohatiner, 1991). High-grade NHL, whether previously treated or not, is much less responsive to IFNα, even at high doses (Leavitt et al., 1987).

High doses of IFNα (i.e. 50 MU three times a week) were found to produce partial (but not complete) responses in about half of patients with mycosis fungoides (Bunn et al., 1986). All patients required dose reduction due to IFNα toxicity. A more recent study has combined etretinate with doses of IFNα between 18 and 36 MU daily; two complete responses were obtained, although IFNα toxicity again resulted in dose reduction (Thestrup-Pedersen et al., 1988). Recently, previously untreated patients have demonstrated a 36% CR rate following up to 18 MU IFNα three times a week, suggesting that early disease is more responsive (Papa et al., 1991).

There are some case reports describing the use of IFNα in advanced Hodgkin's disease, but the agent is not consistently effective.

Chronic lymphatic leukaemia (CLL) Early reports suggesting that CLL is generally unresponsive to IFNα have been borne out (Talpaz et al., 1987a). However, it now appears that early stage disease can respond to 3 MU three times a week, with a fall in circulating lymphocyte count during IFNα therapy (Rozman et al., 1988), but counts generally return to pretreatment levels once treatment is stopped. Our experience is that the lymphocyte count can begin to rise during IFNα therapy, and this may relate to IFNα antibodies (Giles et al., 1990). Other groups have not observed progression during therapy (Ziegle-Heitbroch et al., 1989). It is not clear whether IFNα will modify the course of this disease.

Essential thrombocythaemia Most cases will maintain a platelet count below $600 \times 10^6/l$ on 3 MU three times a week, although daily dosing is usually required to achieve the initial fall in count (Giles et al., 1988). Symptoms and thromboembolic events can also be reduced with IFNα therapy (Gisslinger et al., 1989). Gugliotta et al. (1987) demonstrated that IFNα therapy reduces both the marrow megakaryocyte count and in vitro megakaryocytopoiesis (CFU-Meg 73 ± 18 before therapy, 29 ± 15 during therapy). This reduction in platelet production is accompanied by an improvement in platelet function, although platelet half-life remains unchanged. The platelet count usually rises again once IFNα is discontinued. Essential thrombocythaemia often affects younger individuals and therapy with IFNα or hydroxyurea poses questions in terms of gonadal function and leukaemic transformation. Therefore, contraceptive advice should not be forgotten, and effects on leukaemogenesis remain to be determined.

Immune thrombocytopenia Steroid-resistant ITP can improve after 12 doses of IFNα (3 MU) – the platelet count rising on cessation of therapy in 69% of cases, 19% achieving a complete response (Proctor et al., 1989).

Patients often respond to IFNα again following relapse. No changes in platelet-associated antibody have been described. The mechanism whereby IFNα acts in ITP is presumably rather different to the agent's antiproliferative effect observed in essential thrombocythaemia.

Pancreatic endocrine tumours Substantial palliation can be achieved in two-thirds of these patients (Erikson *et al.*, 1986). In particular, patients with Werner–Morrison syndrome experience cessation of diarrhoea and flushing. The carcinoid syndrome may improve in a similar manner (Oberg and Eriksson, 1991).

AIDS-related Kaposi's sarcoma Krown's initial report (Krown *et al.*, 1983) gave an overall response rate of 38%. Several studies have now shown that such response rates require good residual immune function and up to 30 MU daily may be required for an optimal response (Fischl, 1991). Tolerance of such regimens is variable, but in the presence of AZT, marrow toxicity is often dose-limiting. Lesions usually recur on cessation of therapy. No effect on survival has yet been observed.

Disorders that are minimally responsive to IFNα

Renal cell carcinoma Metastatic disease involving lung, nodes or bone can respond to IFNα at doses of 18 to 36 MU three times a week, in 21% of cases (Fossa *et al.*, 1991). These authors suggest IFNα is the systemic treatment of choice in this situation, although toxicities may overshadow such responses.

Malignant melanoma Although an occasional CR is observed, most studies report less than 20% response rates (Dorval *et al.*, 1986). Predictably, patients with low tumour burdens seem to respond best, and IFNα may find a place in combination with other cytokines or as an adjuvant during cytotoxic therapies.

Myelodysplasia The majority of MDS patients treated with IFNα demonstrate a worsening of their cytopenias, but infection risk does not deteriorate (Galvani *et al.*, 1988a; Elias *et al.*, 1987). Occasionally a patient will demonstrate a reduction in a marrow leukaemic clone, but predicting such rare responses is difficult and does not merit using IFNα in MDS in general (Galvani *et al.*, 1987).

Myelofibrosis IFNα can reduce fibroblast growth and potentially fibrosis (Galvani and Cawley, 1990). However, IFNα therapy has no overall benefit in this disease for most patients (Gastle *et al.*, 1988). Occasional reductions in spleen size and transfusion requirements have been reported with IFNα, but this is unusual (Wickramsinghe *et al.*, 1987).

Acute leukaemia The use of IFNα as a maintenance arm of the British MRC AML XI trial is an attempt to eradicate minimal residual disease. IFNα has little benefit during induction.

IFNα IN VIRAL DISORDERS

Chronic hepatitis B IFNα production is defective in this disorder (Davis and Hoofnagle, 1986). Administering 5 MU three times a week can reduce viral replication and ablate the HBe antigen with the appearance of HBe antibody in one-third of patients (Hoofnagle *et al.*, 1988). Histological improvement may be optimal at 10 MU/m^2 three times a week for three months (Brook *et al.*, 1989), and improvements may persist following cessation of therapy. Poor responders can be predicted by low ALT and high HBV-DNA levels, although higher doses of IFNα in the latter group may improve responsiveness (Herzenberg, 1991). It has been suggested that induction of 2'5'A synthetase may indicate a better response to IFNα, but this remains to be substantiated. The relationship of steroid and IFNα therapy needs further definition.

Chronic hepatitis C Liver histology and transaminase activity can be improved with 3 MU three times a week for 6 months (Davis *et al.*, 1989; Di Bisceglie *et al.*, 1989). However, relapse within six months of stopping IFNα is common, and thus low-dose therapy may need to be given for a prolonged period. With the introduction of routine screening for hepatitis C for blood donors, these findings may have major public health and financial implications.

Human papilloma virus This group of viruses produce recurrent laryngeal papillomatosis (RLP) and condylomata accuminata. IFNα produces dramatic improvements in the distressing symptoms of RLP, but therapy needs to be continued to avoid recurrence (McCabe and Clark, 1983). Although systemic and local IFNα can improve condylomata, this has not gained widespread enthusiasm (Gall *et al.*, 1983).

HIV A daily dose of 3 MU of IFNα has been shown to reduce, and occasionally completely suppress, plasma HIV and p24 antigen in humans (Kovacs *et al.*, 1989). Higher doses may achieve a better effect but also retard the beneficial effect of AZT on the CD4 count (Fischl, 1991). Carefully conducted trials of combination antiretroviral therapy need to be performed to establish long-term benefits.

Rhinovirus Intranasal IFNα may be useful prophylaxis for immunosuppressed individuals but seems hardly justified on a cost–benefit analysis for the general public (Douglas, 1986).

CONCLUSIONS AND FUTURE TRENDS

Whether IFNα proves to be superior to other treatments in HCL and CGL remains to be proven, however, it is clear that the agent can modify these diseases in a manner that is different from conventional therapies. Such antitumour activity is probably antiproliferative in its nature. In myeloma, IFNα may prolong plateau phase. IFNα has yet to find its role in the management of NHL. The role of IFNα in solid tumours will probably be as adjuvant and/or palliative therapy and may be in combination with other 'biological response modifiers'. The possibility of modifying chronic hepatitis may greatly expand the use of IFNα, especially now that hepatitis C testing is becoming widespread.

REFERENCES

Alimena G, Morra E, Lazarino M et al. (1988). Interferon α 2b as therapy for chronic myeloid leukaemia: a study of 82 patients treated with intermittent or daily administration. Blood. 72, 642–7.

Allan NC and Shepherd PCA (1987). Treatment of chronic myeloid leukaemia. In: Chronic myeloid leukaemia, ed. Goldman JM, 1031–54. London: Balliere Tindall.

Anonymous (1980). Interferon nomenclature. Nature. 286, 10.

Brook MO, Petrovic L, McDonald JA et al. (1989). Histological improvement after anti-viral treatment for chronic hepatitis B infection. J Hepatol. 8, 208–25.

Broxmeyer HE, Lu L, Platzer E et al. (1983). Comparative analysis of the influences of human α, β and γ interferons on CFU-GEMM, BFU-E and CFU-GM progenitor cells. J Immunol. 131, 1300–5.

Bunn PA, Ihde DC and Foon KA (1986). The role of interferonα2a in the therapy of cutaneous T-cell lymphoma. Cancer. 57, 1689–95.

Celis JE (1987). Major proteins induced and down regulated by interferons in human cultured cells: identification of a unique set of proteins induced by Interferonα in epithelial, fibroblast and lymphoid cells. Leukaemia. 1, 800–13.

Chebath J, Benech P, Revel M and Vigneron M (1987). Constitutive expression of 2'5'A synthetase confers resistance to picornavirus infection. Nature. 330, 587–8.

Constanzi JJ, Cooper MR, Scarffe JH et al. (1985). Phase II study of recombinant interferon-α in resistant multiple myeloma. J Clin Oncol. 3, 654–9.

Cordingley FT, Bianchi A, Hoffbrand AV et al. (1989). TNF as an autocrine factor for B cell malignancies. Lancet, i, 969–71.

Dadmarz R, Evans T, Secher D, Marshall N and Cawley JC (1987). Hairy-cells possess more Interferon-α receptors than other lymphoid cell types. Leukaemia. 1, 357–61.

Davis GL and Hoofnagle JH (1986). Interferon in viral hepatitis: role in pathogenesis and treatment. Hepatology. 6, 1038–41.

Davis GR, Balat LA, Schiff ER *et al.* (1989). Treatment of chronic hepatitis C with recombinant interferon-α. *N Engl J Med.* **321**, 1501–6.

De Mel WCP, Hoffbrand AV, Giles F *et al.* (1990). Interferon-alpha for haematological malignancies: correlation between in vivo induction of 2'5'oligoadenylate synthetase and clinical response. *Br J Haematol.* **74**, 452–6.

Di Bisceglie AM, Martin P, Kessianides C *et al.* (1989). Recombinant interferon-α for chronic hepatitis C. *N Engl J Med.* **321**, 1506–10.

Dorval T, Palangie T, Jouve M *et al.* (1986). Clinical phase II trial of IFNα in metastatic malignant melanoma. *Cancer.* **58**, 215–8.

Douglas RG (1986). The common cold-relief at last? *N Engl J Med.* **314**, 114–5.

Dowding C, Guo AP, Osterholz J *et al.* (1991). Interferon-α overrides the deficient adhesion of CML progenitor cells to bone marrow stromal cells. *Blood.* **78**, 499–505.

Duncombe AS, Heslop HE, Turner M *et al.* (1989). Autocrine production of TNF inhibits CML growth – a mechanism for chronicity. *Br J Haematol.* **71**, 169.

Ebsworth N, Taylor-Papadimitriou J and Rosengurt F (1984). Cyclic AMP does not mediate inhibition of DNA synthesis by interferon in mouse Swiss 3T3 cells. *J Cell Physiol.* **120**, 146–50.

Einat M, Resnitsky D and Kimchi A (1985). Close link between reduction of c-myc expression by interferon and GO/G1 arrest. *Nature.* **313**, 597–600.

Elias L, Hoffman R, Boswell S, Tensen L and Bonnem EM (1987). A trial of recombinant Interferon-α in the myelodysplastic syndromes. *Leukaemia.* **2**, 105–10.

Erikson B, Oberg K, Alm G *et al.* (1986). Treatment of malignant endocrine pancreatic tumours with human leukocyte interferon. *Lancet.* **ii**, 1307–8.

Fellous A, Ginsberg I and Lattauer UZ (1982). Modulation of tubulin mRNA levels by interferon in human lymphoblastoid cells. *EMBO J.* **7**, 835–9.

Fischl MA (1991) Antiviral therapy in AIDS related Kaposi's sarcoma. *Am J Med.* **90 (Suppl. 4a)**, 18–21.

Fossa SD, Lien HH and Lindegaard M (1991). Effect of recombinant interferon-α a bone metasteses and renal cell carcinoma. *N Engl J Med.* **324**, 633–4.

Freund M, Wussow PV, Diedrich H *et al.* (1989). Recombinant IFNα in chronic myelogenous leukaemia: dose dependency of response and frequency of neutralising antibodies. *Brit J Haematol.* **72**, 350–356.

Fujiyama Y and Pattengale PK (1985). Characterisation of NK cells in patients with chronic myeloid leukaemia. In: *Mechanisms of cytotoxicity of NK cells*, ed. Hebermann RB and Callewaert DM, 521–42. London: Academic Press.

Gall SA, Hughes CE and Troffater K (1983). Interferon-α for therapy of condylomata acuminata. *Am J Obstet Gynecol.* **153**, 157–63.

Galton JE, Bedford P, Scott JE, Brand CM and Nethersell ABW (1989). Antibodies to lymphoblastoid interferon. *Lancet.* **ii**, 572–3.

Galvani DW and Cawley JC (1989). Mechanism of action of interferon-α in CGL: evidence for preferential inhibition of late progenitors. *Br J Haematol.* **73**, 475–9.

Galvani DW and Cawley JC (1990). The effect of interferon-α in human long-term bone marrow cultures. *Leuk Res.* **14**, 525–32.

Galvani DW, Nethersell ABW, Bottomley J and Cawley JC (1987). Interferon in myelodysplasia. *Br J Haematol.* **66**, 145–6.

Galvani DW, Nethersell ABW and Cawley JC (1988a). Interferon-α in myelodysplasia: clinical observations and effects on NK cells. *Leuk Res.* **12**, 257–62.

Galvani DW, Owens W, Nethersell ABW and Cawley JC (1988b). The beneficial effects of interferon-α in CGL are probably not mediated by NK cells. *Br J Haematol.* **71**, 233–7.

Gastle G, Lang A, Huber C *et al.* (1988). Interferon-α for idiopathic myelofibrosis. *Lancet.* **i**, 765–6.

Giles FJ, Singer CRJ, Gray AG *et al.* (1988). Interferon-α for essential thrombocytopenia. *Lancet.* **ii**, 70–2.

Giles FJ, Worman CP, Gaffar RA *et al.* (1990). Early results of Roferon treatment of chronic lymphoid leukaemia. *Br J Haematol.* **74 (Suppl. 1)**, 31.

Gisslinger H, Ludwig H, Linkesch W *et al.* (1989). Long-term interferon-α therapy for thrombocytosis in myeloproliferative diseases. *Lancet.* **i**, 634–7.

Glaspy JA, Baldwin GC, Robertson PA *et al.* (1988). Therapy for neutropenia in hairy-cell leukaemia with recombinant G-CSF. *Ann Int Med.* **109**, 789–95.

Greasey AA, Vitt CR, Herst C *et al.* (1988). Functional properties of proteins coded by three human interferon genes and a pseudogene. *Cancer Res.* **48**, A63–70.

Griffiths SD and Cawley JC (1987). The beneficial effects of α-interferon in hairy-cell leukaemia are not attributable to NK cell mediated cytotoxocity. *Leukaemia.* **1**, 372–376.

Griffiths SD and Cawley JC (1988). Interferon-α and LAK cell activity in hairy-cell leukaemia. *Leukaemia.* **2**, 377–81.

Griffiths SD and Cawley JC (1989). The effects of cytokines, including IL–2, IL-4 and IL-6, in hairy cell proliferation/differentiation. *Leukaemia.* **4**, 337–40.

Griffiths SD and Cawley JC (1991). Monocyte/macrophages stimulate hairy-cell proliferation. *Leukaemia and Lymphoma.* **4**, 325–30.

Griffiths SD, Galvani DW and Cawley JC (1989). The Interferons. In: *Immunotherapy of Disease*, ed. Hamblin TJ, 43–70. London: Kluwer Press.

Grossenberg SE, Taylor JL and Kusheyer VM (1989). Interferon receptors and their role in interferon action. *Experimentia.* **45**, 508–10.

Gugliotta A, Macchi S and Catani L (1987). Evaluation of thrombopoiesis in essential thromobcytosis before and after interferon-α therapy. *Throm and Haem.* **58**, 481–4.

Harada H, Fujifa T, Hiyamoto M *et al.* (1989). Structurally similar but functionally distinct factors IRF1 and IRF2 bind to the same regulatory elements of Interferon and Interferon inducible genes. *Cell.* **58**, 729–33.

Herzenberg H (1991). Interferon-α for chronic hepatitis B. *N Engl J Med.* **324**, 493–4.

Hoofnagle JH, Peters M, Mullen KD and Jones EA (1988). Randomised controlled trial of interferon-α in chronic hepatitis B. *Gastro.* **95**, 1318–25.

Kimchi A (1981). Increased levels of interferon induced (2'5') oligoadenylate synthetase in mature T-lymphocytes and in differentiated Friend erythroleukaemic cells. *J Interferon Res.* **1**, 559–69.

Knight E, Anton ED, Fahey D, Friedland BK and Joual GJ (1985). Interferon-α regulates c-myc expression in Daudi cells at the post-transcriptional level. *Proc Natl Acad Sci USA.* **82**, 1151–4.

Kovacs J, Deytor L, Davey R *et al.* (1989). Combined AZT and interferon-α in Kaposis sarcoma and AIDS. *Ann Int Med.* **111**, 280–7.

Kraut EH, Bouroncle BA and Grever MR (1986). Low dose deoxycoformycin in the treatment of hairy-cell leukaemia. *Blood.* **68**, 1119–22.

Krown S, Real FX, Cunningham-Rundle S *et al.* (1983). Preliminary observations on the effect of recombinant interferon-α in homosexual men with Kaposi's sarcoma. *N Eng J Med.* **308**, 1071–6.

Kurzrock R, Talpaz M, Kantarjian H and Gutterman JU (1987).Therapy of chronic myelogenous leukaemia with recombinant interferon gamma. *Blood.* **70**, 943–47.

Leavitt RD, Ratanatharathorn V, Ozer H *et al.* (1987). Alfa-2b interferon in the treatment of Hodgkin's and non-Hodgkin's disease. *Sem Oncol.* **14**, 18–23.

Ludwig H, Cortelezzi A, Scheithauer W *et al.* (1986). Recombinant Interferon-α2c versus polychemotherapy (VMCP) for the treatment of multiple myeloma: a prospective randomized trial. *Eur J Can Clin Oncol.* **22**, 1111–16.

Mandelli F, Avvisati G, Amadori S *et al.* (1990). Maintenance treatment with recombinant interferon-α in patients with multiple myeloma responding to conventional induction chemotherapy. *N Engl J Med.* **322**, 1430–4.

McCabe BF and Clark KF (1983). Interferon-alpha and laryngeal papillomatosis. *Ann Otol Rhin Laryngol.* **92**, 2–7.

McDonald R (1987). Interferons as mediators of psychiatric morbidity. An investigation in a trial of interferon in hepatitis B carriers. *Lancet.* **ii**, 1175–8.

McKinnon S, Hows JM and Goldman JM (1990). In vitro analysis of graft versus leukaemia activity following BMT for CGL. *Br J Haematol.* **74 (Suppl. 1)**, 14.

Mehmet H, Morris CME, Taylor-Papadimitriou J and Rozengurt E (1987). Interferon-α inhibition of DNA synthesis in Swiss 3T3 cells: Dissociation from protein kinase C activation. *Biochem Biophys Res Comm.* **145**, 1026–32.

Morgensen MF, Uze G and Eid P (1989). The cellular receptor for Interferon-α. *Experimentia.* **45**, 500–8.

Oberg K and Eriksson B (1991). The role of interferons in the management of carcinoid tumours. *Br J Haematol.* **79 (Suppl. 1)**, 74–7.

O'Connell MJ, Colgen JP, Oken MM *et al.* (1987). Clinical trial of recombinant interferon as initial therapy for favourable histology non-Hodgkin's lymphoma. *J Clin Oncol.* **4**, 128–36.

127

Oken HM, Kyle RA, Kay NE *et al.* (1990). Interferon-α in the treatment of refractory multiple myeloma: An Eastern Co-operative Group Study. *Leuk and Lymph.* **1**, 95–100.

Oken MM, Kyle RA, Griepp PR *et al.* (1988). Alternating cycles of VBMCP with interferon (rIFN-α2) in the treatment of multiple myeloma. *Proc Am Soc Clin Onc.* **7**, 868a.

Papa G, Tura S, Mandelli ML *et al.* (1991). Is interferon alpha in cutaneous T-cell lymphoma a treatment of choice? *Br J Haematol.* **79** (**Suppl. 1**), 48–51.

Pelus LM, Ottmann OG and Nocka KH (1988). Synergistic inhibition of human CFU-GU progenitor cells by prostaglan E, interferons and TNF. *J Immunol.* **140**, 479–84.

Pfeffer LM, Strulovici B and Saltiel AR (1990). Interferon-α selectively activates the β-isoform of protein kinase C through phaphatidylcholine hydrolysis. *Proc Natl Acad Sci USA.* **87**, 6537–41.

Piro LD, Carrera CJ, Carson DA and Beutler E (1990). Lasting remissions in hairy-cell leukaemia induced by a single infusion of 2-chlorodeoxyadenosine. *N Eng J Med.* **322**, 1117–21.

Proctor S, Jackson GH, Carey P *et al.* (1989). Improvement in platelet counts in steroid unresponsive ITP following short course recombinant alpha2b interferon. *Blood.* **74**, 1894–7.

Resnitsky D, Yarden A, Zipori D and Kimchi A (1986). Autocrine-related interferon controls c-myc suppression and growth arrest during haemopoietic cell differentiation. *Cell.* **46**, 31–40.

Rohatiner AZS (1991). Interferon alpha in lymphoma. *Br J Haematol.* **79** (**Suppl. 1**), 26–9.

Rosenblum MG, Maxwell BL, Talpaz M *et al.* (1986). In vivo sensitivity and resistance of CML cells to IFNα: correlation with receptor binding and induction of 2'5'oligoadenylate synthetase. *Cancer Res.* **46**, 4848–52.

Rossi GB (1985). Interferon in cell differentiation. In: *Interferon 6*, ed. Gresser I, 31–68. London: Academic Press.

Rozman C, Monserrat E, Vinolas N *et al.* (1988). Recombinant interferon-α in the treatment of B-CLL in early stages. *Blood.* **71**, 1295–8.

Rubinstein M and Orchansky P (1986). The Interferon Receptors. *CRC Crit Rev Biochem.* **21**, 249–75.

Samuel C, Duncan R, Knutsen G and Hershey W (1984). Mechanism of interferon action. *J Biol Chem.* **259**, 13451–7.

Schtalrid M, Blick M, Kurzrock R *et al.* (1989). Variable expression of 2'5'A synthetase and HLA-B genes in CML patients treated with interferon. *Exp Haematol.* **17**, 609.

Silverman RH (1982). The ppp(A2'p)nA and protein kinase systems in wild-type and interferon-resistant Daudi cells. *Eur J Biochem.* **126**, 333–41.

Sreevalsan T (1980). Differential effect of interferon on DNA synthesis, 2-deoxyglucose uptake and ornithine decarboxylase activity in 3T3 cells stimulated with polypeptide growth factors. *J Cell Physiol.* **104**, 1–9.

Staeheli P and Haller O (1987). Interferon induced Mx protein: A mediator of cellular resistance to influenza virus. In: *Interferon 8*, ed. Gresser I, 2–24. London: Academic Press.

Steis RG, Foon KA and Longo DL (1987). Current and future uses of recombinant interferon-α in the treatment of low-grade non-Hodgkin's lymphoma. *Cancer.* **59**, 658–63.

Steis RG, Smith JW, Urba WJ *et al.* (1988). Resistance to recombinant interferon 2α in hairy-cell leukaemia associated with neutralising antibodies. *N Eng J Med.* **318**, 1409–13.

Strife A and Clarkson B (1988). Biology of chronic granulocytic leukaemia: Is discordant maturation the primary defect? *Sem Haematol.* **25**, 1–19.

Talpaz M, Rosenblum R, Kurzrock R *et al.* (1987a). Clinical and laboratory changes induced by interferon-α in chronic lymphocytic leukaemia. *Am J Haematol.* **24**, 341–50.

Talpaz M, Kantarjian HM, McCredie KB *et al.* (1987b). Clinical investigation of IFNα in chronic myeloid leukaemia. *Blood.* **69**, 1280–8.

Tamm I, Lin SL, Pfeffer ZM and Sehgal PC (1987). Interferons α and β as cellular regulatory molecules. In: *Interferon 9*, ed. Gresser I, 14–74. London: Academic Press.

Tanaka M, Kimura K and Yoshida (1987). Inhibition of mammalian DNA polymerases by recombinant Interferon α and γ. *Cancer Res.* **47**, 5971–4.

Taylor-Papadimitriou J and Rozengurt E (1985). Interferons as regulators of cell growth and differentiation. In: *Interferons: their impact in biology and medicine*, ed. J Taylor-Papadimitriou 81–98. Oxford: Oxford University Press.

Thestrup-Pedersen K, Hammer R, Kaltoft K, Sogaard H and Zachariae H (1988). Treatment of mycosis fungoides with recombinant interferon-α alone and in combination with etretinate. *Br J Dermatol.* **118**, 811–8.

Tovey MG, Gresser I, Rochette-Egly C *et al.* (1982). Indomethacin and aspirin do not inhibit the antiviral or antiproliferative effects of interferon. *J Gen Virol.* **63**, 505–8.

von Wussow PV, Pralle H, Hochkeppel HK *et al.* (1991a). Effective natural Interferon-α therapy in recombinant interferon-α-resistant patients with hairy cell leukaemia. *Blood.* **78**, 38–43.

von Wussow PV, Jakschies D, Freund M *et al.* (1991b). Treatment of anti-recombinant interferon-alpha2 antibody positive CML patients with natural interferon-alpha. *Br J Haematol.* **78**, 210–16.

Wickramsinghe SN, Peert S and Gill DS (1987). Interferon-α in primary idiopathic myelofibrosis. *Lancet.* **i**, 1524–5.

Williams BRG and Fish EN (1985). Interferon and viruses: In vitro studies. In: *Interferons: their impact in biology and medicine*, ed. J Taylor-Papadimitriou, 40-60. Oxford: Oxford University Press.

Worman C, Catovsky D, Bevan PC *et al.* (1985). Interferon-α is effective in hairy-cell leukaemia. *Br J Haematol.* **60**, 759–63.

Yap WH, Teo TS, McCoy E and Tan YH (1986). Rapid and transient rise indiacylglycerol concentration in Daudi cells exposed to interferon. *Proc Natl Acad Sci USA.* **83**, 7765–9

Ziegle-Heitbroch HWL, Schlag R, Flige D and Thiel E (1989). Favourable response of early stage B-CLL patients to interferon-α. *Blood.* **73**, 1426–30.

9

INTERFERON-GAMMA

R. KURZROCK

INTRODUCTION

The similarities between interferon-α (IFNα) and β make it very likely that their genes diverged from a common ancestor over 200 million years ago. However, if IFNγ originated from the same common ancestor gene, it must have done so much earlier, as it is structurally and biologically quite different from IFNα and β.

MOLECULAR BIOLOGY

Unlike IFNα, only a single gene has been identified for IFNγ. This gene is considered molecularly distinct from IFNα and IFNβ, and has only about 12% amino acid homology to IFNα. The IFNγ gene has four exons, and regulatory elements reminiscent of those for IL-2 and the p55 (*Tac*) chain of the IL-2 receptor.

IFNγ is considerably less conserved between species than IFNβ, which is in turn less conserved than the IFNα family. This suggests that there are stronger constraints on the IFNα than on the IFNγ proteins. The activities of the interferons show, to variable degrees, species specificity. Some human IFNαs are active on mouse cells while others, as well as IFNβ and IFNγ, are not.

PHYSICOCHEMICAL CHARACTERISTICS

There is evidence for only one IFNγ gene in all species analysed. In humans, the gene is localized on chromosome 12 and codes for a single polypeptide made up of a signal peptide of 20 amino acids and a mature protein of 146

131

amino acids. The protein has a molecular weight of 17 kDa. It appears that the mature human IFNγ protein has no cysteine residues and it follows that disulphide bonds do not exist. The IFNγ molecule contains two potential glycosylation sites. Depending on the carbohydrate groups attached, IFNγ can be secreted as a glycoprotein with molecular weights varying from 20–25 kDa in man. The presence of carbohydrate moieties on IFNγ affects its biochemical but not its functional properties. Glycosidase treatment of IFNγ does not reduce its antiviral activity, affect the interaction with specific antibody, or change its target cell specificity (Ijzermans and Marquet, 1989) Human IFNγ contains an acid labile Asp-Pro bond between positions 2 and 3. Treatment at pH 2.3 breaks this bond with subsequent loss of IFNγ's antiviral activity.

Target analysis suggests that the IFNγ functional unit is a tetramer, although gel filtration studies indicate that the natural state is a dimer. Studies of the recombinant molecule indicate that removal of four C-terminal amino acids has minimal consequences, whereas deletion of 19 C-terminal residues results in a 1000-fold decrease in antiviral and antiproliferative activities (Zoon, 1987).

IFNγ PRODUCTION

The gene for IFNγ can be stimulated by in vitro exposure to non-specific mitogens, antigens, or interleukin-2. After such stimulation, human T4+ (helper) cells, T8+ (suppressor) cells and natural killer cells secrete IFNγ (Kasahara et al., 1983; Handa et al., 1983). Until recently, IFNγ was considered the exclusive product of these cells, but it now appears that in vitro-triggered alveolar macrophages from healthy volunteers can also generate IFNγ (Nugent et al., 1985). However, it is mainly the T4+ cell derived from peripheral blood or serous cavities that produces IFNγ after exposure to a soluble microbial antigen. Although interleukin-2 is an important stimulus for the IFNγ gene, selected microbial antigens can also induce T4+ cell IFNγ production by an auxiliary mechanism that is largely independent of interleukin-2. T cell proliferation is not necessarily required for IFNγ generation.

Once stimulated by mitogen or antigen, the production of IFNγ by activated T cells occurs rapidly, with full expression of transcripts and protein by 6 h. Peak IFNγ levels are generally observed by 48 to 72 h and in vitro production may continue for as long as 8 days.

The immune circuitry that culminates in IFNγ production is intertwined with that of other cytokines. As mentioned earlier, interleukin-2 stimulates IFNγ production; conversely, IFNγ may, by inducing interleukin-1, indirectly stimulate interleukin-2 production. Further, responsiveness to interleukin-2 is increased by IFNγ because of the induction of interleukin-2 receptors on T cells. Finally, interleukin-1, secreted by IFNγ-triggered macrophages, may act synergistically with interleukin-2 to augment IFNγ secretion (Le *et al.*, 1986).

IFNγ RECEPTOR

All human cells tested so far carry a receptor for IFNγ, characterized by high affinity and specificity to the ligand. The observed species specificity normally associated with IFNγ seems to be dependent on the interaction of the molecule with the cell membrane receptor.

The IFNγ receptor is a single chain glycoprotein with an apparent molecular mass of 90 kDa. It is mainly *N*-glycosylated; the carbohydrate moiety contributes about 17 kDa to the receptor protein molecular weight and is not essential for receptor-binding activity.

The gene for the IFNγ receptor is located on chromosome 6. According to the cDNA sequence, the receptor is a protein of 489 amino acids. In addition to the internal signal peptide (amino acids 1–17), hydropathy analysis of the translated sequences reveals a hydrophobic domain in the middle of the molecule (amino acids 246–66), compatible with a transmembrane anchoring region. Experiments with monoclonal antibodies indicate that the *N*-terminus of the IFNγ receptor is extracellular (Garotta *et al.*, 1989).

Binding of IFNγ to its receptor is followed by receptor-mediated endocytosis and ligand degradation, but it is not clear if IFNγ needs to be internalized to exert its biological effects (Branca *et al.*, 1982).

Experiments with antireceptor antibodies suggest that activation of the receptor may be sufficient to initiate transmembranous and intracellular signalling. However, if IFNγ is introduced into the cell via liposomes, thus bypassing the receptor, biologic activity is also observed.

BIOLOGICAL ACTIVITIES

IFNγ is not primarily an antiviral agent, although it does have antiviral activity. Under physiological conditions, IFNγ is produced much later during the course of viral infection as compared to IFNα or β. Further, viruses differ

Table 9.1. *Immunological activities of IFN-γ* *

Cellular target	Biological effect
Macrophage	Induces expression of MHC Class II antigens, Fc receptors, and Integrin receptors (Mac-1, CR3, LFA-1) Induces IL-1 and TNF synthesis Activates respiratory burst and microbicidal and tumoricidal activity
T lymphocytes	Induces maturation of cytotoxic T cells Inhibits T-suppressor maturation Increases ICAM-1 expression Enhances proliferation of T cells and IL-2 release
B lymphocytes	Differential control of immunoglobulin isotype synthesis
Endothelial cells	Induces MHC Class II antigens, ICAM-1 and release of chemotactic factors
Epithelial cells	Induces MHC Class II antigens and ICSM-I
NK cells	Enhances cytotoxicity

* Adapted from Garotta *et al.*, 1989.

in their sensitivity to IFNα, β, or IFNγ, with some viruses being more strongly inhibited by interferons-α and β, whereas other viruses are more sensitive to IFNγ. IFNγ also exerts in vitro antiproliferative effects. In some tumour cell lines, this activity may be more pronounced than that exerted by IFNα or β, though IFNα is a much more potent antitumour agent in the clinic. The most potent effects of IFNγ are in the arena of immune regulation.

Immunomodulation

All interferons have profound effects on the immune system; IFNγ, in particular, is a pivotal, endogenous immunoregulator (Table 9.1). The key role of interferons in immunity is underscored by the observation that nearly

Table 9.2. *Non-viral pathogens susceptible to IFN-γ activated monocyte/macrophage effects* *

Type	Pathogen
Protozoa	*Toxoplasma hondii, Leishmania (donovani, major* and *mexicana), Trypanosoma cruzi, Entamoeba histolytica, Plasmodium falciparum*
Helminth	*Schistosoma mansoni*
Bacteria	*Listeria monocytogenes, Salmonella typhimurium, Legionella pneumophilia, Mycobacterium tuberculosis*
Fungi	*Histoplasma capsulatum, Candida albicans, Candida parapsilosis, Cryptococcus neoformans, Blastomyces dermatiditis*
Chlamydia	*Chlamydia psittaci, Chlamydia trachomatis*
Rickettsia	*Rickettsia prowazekii, Rickettsia coronii, Rickettsia tsutsugamushi*

* Adapted from Nathan, 1986.

all measurable immune functions can be altered by these molecules. Consequently, there has been tremendous interest in exploitation of IFN-triggered immunomodulation for tumoricidal and microbicidal purposes.

Monocyte/macrophage activation It has long been appreciated that the function of these phagocytes is not static, but rather can be directed down a variety of disparate paths. The macrophage, after entering the tissues, often becomes a relatively inert resident cell, unless confronted with one or more stimulatory signals. Although in some experiments, IFNα and β affect monocyte/macrophage functions, high concentrations are required, suggesting that these molecules are unlikely to act as physiological regulators of these cells. In contrast, IFNγ is a powerful stimulant of monocytes/macrophages both in vitro and in vivo in humans (Murray, 1988).

A wealth of studies link IFNγ with the two expressions of monocyte/macrophage activation most relevant to host defence – enhanced antimicrobial activity and tumour cell cytotoxicity. IFNγ, released by antigen-triggered T4+ cells, converts quiescent macrophages to efficient microbicidal and tumoricidal phagocytes capable of killing or inhibiting diverse human neoplastic cells and intracellular pathogens (Nathan, 1986 – see Table 9.2).

IFNγ participates in the eradication of neoplastic cells and invasive organisms by evoking multiple monocyte/macrophage-related processes: (1) release of toxic oxygen intermediates such as hydrogen peroxide (oxygen-independent process); (2) degradation of extracellular tryptophan (oxygen-independent process); (3) expression of monocyte/macrophage Fc receptors with which opsonized organisms can interact; (4) release of lysosomal enzymes; (5) activation of antibody-dependent cellular cytoxicity; (6) phagocytosis, and (7) expression of HLA-DR, a class II major histocompatibility complex molecule required by monocyte/macrophages when they present antigen to helper T cells.

Mononuclear phagocytes bear a distinct receptor for IFNγ on their surface, and engagement of this receptor may be critical before IFNγ can exert its influence. The human monocyte derived macrophage is a quiescent cell that usually requires at least 12-24 h, and up to 72 h, of in vitro exposure to IFNγ before showing optimal expression of the activated state. The activated phenotype is a relatively transient phenomenon and wanes within 2 to 3 days after removal of IFNγ. In contrast, if the fresh peripheral blood monocyte, a cell already intrinsically active in antimicrobial and respiratory burst capacity (H_2O_2 release), is treated with IFNγ, the results are quite different. A comparatively brief exposure (6–24 h) to relatively low concentrations of recombinant IFNγ induces persistent activation for up to 5–7 days in the absence of further treatment (Nathan, 1986).

The mononuclear phagocytes antimicrobial mechanisms are both oxygen-dependent (respiratory burst-dependent) and oxygen-independent. Treatment of the resting macrophage with IFNγ increases the capacity to release toxic oxygen intermediates, including H_2O_2 (Nakagawara et al., 1982). Macrophages are highly sensitive to IFNγ, requiring only 6 pm/ml/10^6 cells to induce oxidative metabolism. Oxygen-independent mechanisms are also stimulated by IFNγ, e.g. enzymatic degradation of extracellular tryptophan and limiting the availability of iron.

Ex vivo experiments on cells obtained from patients with cancer, leprosy and AIDS have shown that exogenously administered IFNγ can also induce monocyte/macrophage activation in humans. In patients with cancer, recombinant IFNγ increases serum lysozyme (Kurzrock et al, 1986c,d), a test that reflects macrophage activity. Further, in these patients, 250 to 500 mcg/m²/day of recombinant IFNγ, given by intramuscular injection, enhanced the antimelanoma tumouricidal activity of blood monocytes (Kleinerman et al., 1986). Higher and lower doses were less effective. However, in another study, intramuscular or subcutaneous injections of only 10 to 100 mcg/m²/day of IFNγ resulted in augmented release of hydrogen peroxide by monocytes derived from individuals suffering from cancer (Maluish *et al.*, 1987) or lepromatous leprosy.

IFNγ can, in addition, inhibit the release, by monocytes, of potentially suppressive prostaglandins; it can also prime mononuclear cells to produce tumour necrosis factor – a cytokine whose macrophage inducing properties are synergistic with those of IFNγ.

The actual interaction between an organism and the macrophage is complex and involves extracellular release of lysosomal enzymes, activation of antibody-mediated cellular toxicity and phagocytosis. Receptors for the Fc portion of IgG are important in the activation of these mononuclear functions since an opsonized organism interacts with macrophage Fc receptors. All three classes of interferon enhance Fc receptors on mononuclear cells, but IFNγ is by far the most potent. IFNγ augmentation of these receptors has been shown to occur in vitro in HL-60, U-937, and K562 cells, as well as in cells derived from normal volunteers, and requires new protein synthesis (Bonnem and Oldham, 1987)

Induction of major histocompatibility complex antigens Interferon causes a 5–10-fold increase in the HLA mRNAs; they increase rapidly and reach a maximum within 4 h of exposure to interferon and they may remain high for 24 h. IFNα, β and γ all stimulate the expression of Class I MHC-associated antigens, but IFNγ is somewhat more efficient. In vitro, the concentrations of IFNα and β1 required for induction of these antigens are in the same range as those necessary for induction of the antiviral state whereas IFNγ induces Class I MHC-associated antigens at much lower concentrations than those needed for inhibition of viral replication. IFNγ also induces these molecules efficiently when used in man (Kurzrock *et al.*, 1986a). The Class I MHC molecules bind non-self antigens and are recognized by cytotoxic T lymphocytes. Therefore, exposure to interferon may make target cells more susceptible to lysis by cytotoxic T cells.

IFNγ also induces Class II MHC antigens such as HLA-DR (Ia antigen) both in vitro and in man. HLA-DR is required by macrophages when they present antigen to helper T cells. In cultured human keratinocytes, HLA-DR is induced within 1–2 days of IFNγ exposure, with maximum expression observed after 4–8 days. IFNγ also effectively induces HLA-DR on both neonatal and adult Langerhans cells, as well as dendritic epidermal cells. The ability of Langerhans cells to function as accessory cells in initiating the immune response is, like that of macrophages, dependent on the expression of Class II HLA antigens. Thus, IFNγ may play a role in regulating skin-associated immune response.

IFNγ stimulates the expression of HLA-DR, HLA-DP and HLA-DQ Class II antigens on cultured human vascular endothelial cells and the adhesion of lymphocytes to the endothelial cells, whereas IFNα does not. The majority of the lymphocytes that adhere are Leu-3+ T cells. The adhesion is obviated by anti-HLA-DR or anti-Leu-3a antibody. Therefore, the interaction of the Leu-3 (T4) receptor with IFNγ-induced DR antigens on the endothelial cell surface may play a central role in the selective adhesion of T4 lymphocytes to vascular endothelium.

IFNγ, but not IFNα or β, is responsible for HLA-DR expression on certain breast cancer, melanoma, osteogenic sarcoma, colorectal cancer and glioma cell lines. However, in SW480 cells, both IFNα and β enhance the expression of Class II antigens. Comparative studies of the effects of interferons on Class II HLA molecules in a melanoma and a lymphoblastoid cell line, as well as in peripheral blood mononuclear cells of human origin, showed that IFNγ markedly increases Class II HLA antigens; IFNβ has a lesser enhancing effect; and IFNα is without effect (Capobionchi et al., 1985).

The mechanisms involved in IFN-related control of MHC antigens have been only partially elucidated. Present evidence supports the existence of at least four conserved, upstream, IFN-responsive, transcriptional regulatory sequences in human MHC Class II genes. Not all of these sequences are shared by MHC Class I genes. One, however, appears to be homologous to the IFN-stimulated response element (ISRE) found upstream of Class I MHC genes. The observation that this ISRE is located further upstream of MHC Class II than of Class I genes has led to the speculation that its importance in regulating Class II genes may be limited, and it may only be involved in the slight IFNα-induced upregulation occasionally noted.

Natural killer cell regulation Natural killer (NK) cells show spontaneous cytotoxic activity against tumour cells and, unlike T cells, do not require the expression of HLA molecules. Contradictory reports regarding the effect of interferons on natural killer cells can be found in the literature. Some investigators have demonstrated reduced susceptibility of target cells to natural killer cell cytotoxicity subsequent to IFNβ treatment. Conversely, human IFNα and IFNγ have been shown to augment NK cell antibody-dependent cellular cytotoxicity as well as direct cytotoxicity against K562 (chronic myelogenous leukaemia blast crisis) cells (Giedlund et al., 1987). The kinetics of the augmentation require only minutes with IFNα and several hours with IFNγ in vitro.

Ex vivo, augmentation of tumoricidal activity has also been documented in cancer patients after injections of recombinant IFNγ (Kurzrock et al., 1986c,d). Much of what IFNγ does may be at the behest of, or in concert with, interleukin-2; these two molecules can, directly or indirectly, stimulate production of each other, and interleukin-2 triggers NK cells. Therefore, the IFNγ/NK cell activation pathway may be a self-amplifying system.

Effects on T cells These are summarized in Table 9.1. IFNα may increase cytotoxic T lymphocyte activity and IFNγ may inhibit generation of these cells in vitro (Welsh *et al.*, 1988). However, by inducing MHC Class I antigens, interferons may also enhance target cell susceptibility to lysis by cytotoxic T lymphocytes. Further, IFNγ also induces monocyte secretion of interleukin-1, which amplifies the production of interleukin-2 and its receptor. Interleukin-2 then influences the generation and activation of various cytotoxic lymphocyte populations capable of lysing tumour cells. The lymphocyte populations include the lymphokine activated killer (LAK) cells (non-MHC-restricted peripheral blood cytotoxic cell population containing subgroups with phenotypic resemblances to T cells and NK cells) and the tumour-infiltrating lymphocytes (TILs).

Effects on B cells IFNα can induce final differentiation to immunoglobulin production, inhibit B cell activation, and influence isotype switching. IFNγ functions as an obligatory early- and late-acting B cell differentiation factor. This activity may be mediated via either direct or indirect mechanisms. Based on experiments with monoclonal B cell lines, Sidman and co-workers (1984) postulated that IFNγ has a direct role in driving the maturation of resting B cells to active immunoglobulin secretion. The indirect mechanism may involve enhancement of antigen processing due to increased expression of MHC Class II molecules on monocytes. However, studies also indicate that IFNγ can inhibit the proliferation of resting B cells that can be stimulated by B cell stimulatory factor-1. Thus, the interaction of IFNγ with B cells may be complex and B cell stimulating factor-1 may act as a reciprocal regulatory agent in B cell responses. Finally, interferon is also implicated in the differential control of isotype expression; it enhances IgG2a synthesis and suppresses IgG1 and IL-4-induced production (Jurado *et al.*, 1989).

Induction of tumour-associated antigens

In vitro, IFNα and IFNγ have been demonstrated to elicit the expression of specific tumour-associated antigens on the surface of tumour cells already expressing the antigen, and to induce their expression on the surface of carcinoma cells not previously expressing the antigen (Murray *et al.*, 1988). The cells studied include lines originating from melanoma and from breast and colon carcinomas. Exploitation of interferon to enhance tumour antigens may therefore prove useful for detection of tumour masses and for improvement of immunotherapy with monoclonal antibodies.

Antiproliferative effects

There is great variability in the sensitivity of various tumour cell lines to the effects of IFNγ, and many lines are more sensitive to IFNγ than to IFNα. Despite this in vitro observation, IFNγ is a weak antitumour agent in cancer patients, especially as compared to IFNα.

Several mechanisms may be involved in the antiproliferative activities of IFNγ. Depending upon the tumour cell line tested, IFNγ may have direct antiproliferative effects mediated through specific membrane receptor binding, and a relationship between the number of cell membrane receptors and the efficacy of IFNγ has been demonstrated (Ucer et al., 1985). In addition, indirect effects mediated through reduction in oncogene (myc) expression have also been postulated.

Antiviral activity

Antiviral activity has been demonstrated for IFNγ, both in vitro and in vivo (Shalaby et al., 1985). Further, IFNγ potentiates the antiviral activities of IFNα and β. Replication of vesicular stomatitis and encephalomyocarditis virus is inhibited more strongly by IFNα/β whereas reovirus and vaccinia virus display more sensitivity to IFNγ (Rubin and Gupta, 1980). Viruses, therefore, have differential sensitivity to the various interferons. Because IFNα and β are released by cells within hours after viral infection (Dianzoni and Baron, 1975) whereas IFNγ is produced later, it appears that IFNα/β act as a first line of defence, secondarily amplified by IFNγ.

Lipid metabolism

There are several lines of evidence suggesting that interferons provide a communication link between the body's host defence and energy storage systems. In this regard, IFNγ is an especially potent regulator of lipid metabolism. In cancer patients, exogenously administered IFNγ inhibits the key enzyme in triglyceride metabolism (lipoprotein lipase) and consequently causes a profound rise in triglyceride and very low density lipoprotein levels (Kurzrock et al., 1986b). Inhibition is probably rendered via a direct effect on enzyme production. Similar metabolic derangements are observed in cachectic tumour-bearing or infected animals. IFNα also modulates lipid pathways, albeit differently from IFNγ: cholesterol levels are lowered, without an effect on triglycerides (Kurzrock *et al.*, 1986b). These observations implicate a role for the interferons, in particular IFNγ, in regulating the human lipid metabolic profile. Secretion of this immune mediator during chronic illness may serve to mobilize energy reserves from adipose cells preferentially for the immune system, and eventually result in the marked wasting diathesis which is a clinical hallmark of cancer.

PHARMACOLOGY OF IFNγ

Native IFNγ is not absorbed after intramuscular administration and has a rapid serum disappearance curve after intravenous bolus injections. Consistent serum antiviral activity can, however, be maintained with continuous intravenous infusions (Gutterman *et al.*, 1984).

Recombinant IFNγ has been studied both in the laboratory and in cancer patients. Importantly, the compound produced by different pharmaceutical industries can vary in its N-terminal sequences and in its specific activity: rIFNγ (Genentech Inc and Biogen Corp), 2×10^7 units/mg; rIFNγ (Schering Corp), 2×10^6 units/mg. Cognizance of these differences and the potential for variability in biologic properties is essential in comparing results of published studies.

Pharmacokinetic evaluation of recombinant IFNγ has been performed. Using an ELISA and a bioassay, recombinant IFNγ (Genetech Inc) has been shown to have a short half-life (30 min) after intravenous bolus injection (Kurzrock *et al.*, 1985); recombinant IFNγ (Biogen S.A.) was found to have a half-life of 0.8–3.5 h (Van der Berg *et al.*, 1985). In contrast to native IFN-γ, 33 to 77% of an intramuscularly administered dose of the recombinant material (Genetech Inc) is absorbed. As with IFNα, prolonged absorption probably occurs. Subcutaneous recombinant IFNγ (Schering Corp) also results in prolonged serum levels and is biologically active (Thompson *et al.*, 1987); however, some investigators have found inconsistent bioavailability, and they suggested that this might compromise the efficacy of subcutaneous injection (Wagstaff *et al.*, 1987).

After administration of maximum tolerated doses of recombinant IFNγ (Genetech Inc), peak serum levels of 5000-10 000 U/ml (intravenous bolus), 60 U/ml (6-h intravenous infusion), undetectable (24-h intravenous infusions), and 200 U/ml (intramuscular), can be achieved (Kurzrock *et al.*, 1991). In these studies, the lower serum concentrations are a result of decreased tolerance and, hence, a lower maximum tolerated dose for 24 h as compared to 6-h and bolus injections. The maximum tolerated dose of intramuscular injections is intermediate. In general, neutralizing antibodies are not found with the use of this material. The observation that high serum concentrations can only be tolerated for very short periods of time, and that prolonged exposure can only be achieved in the presence of low serum concentrations, should be taken into account when planning in vitro modelling studies of recombinant IFNγ.

ENDOGENOUS IFNγ AND DISEASE

Overproduction Although IFNγ is seldom seen in the serum of healthy individuals, it has been detected in tissue and/or serum derived from patients with various infectious and inflammatory diseases. For instance, in sarcoidosis, an inflammatory disorder characterized by increased number and activity of T4+ cells, the granulomatous areas of the lungs and lymph nodes contain IFNγ. In addition, tissue IFNγ has now been demonstrated immunocytochemically in several other inflammatory diseases – tuberculosis, rheumatoid arthritis, polymyositis and subacute thyroiditis. Biologically active IFNγ can also be discerned in vesicle fluid of patients with Herpes simplex infection, in the serum of patients with *Plasmodium falciparum* malaria, and in the cerebrospinal fluid of victims of viral encephalitis, meningitis and multiple sclerosis. IFNγ has also been implicated in type I diabetes, systemic lupus erythematosus, Schwartzman's reaction, delayed hypersensitivity, and marrow transplant rejection. Finally, Zoumbos and co-workers (1985) have implicated endogenously produced IFNγ as the mediator of haematopoietic suppression in aplastic anaemia; however, more recently, this finding has been disputed by Torok-Storb and colleagues (Torok-Storb *et al.*, 1987).

Underproduction There are many examples of acquired defects in IFNγ secretion, though not all instances correlate with increased vulnerability to opportunistic infections. These defects can reflect an inadequate response to mitogen, a global T cell failure to respond to antigen, or the inability of T4-

Table 9.3. *Disorders with defects in IFNγ production**

Type	Disorder
Autoimmune	SLE, rheumatoid arthritis
Infectious	Fulminant viral hepatitis, viral meningoencephalitis, condylomata acuminata, orolabial herpes simplex, CMV, malaria, leprosy, leishmaniasis, tuberculosis, filariasis
Immune deficiency	AIDS, transplantation (renal, cardiac and marrow), hyper-IgE syndrome
Cancer	Lymphoma, intracranial, lymphocytic leukaemia (acute and chronic)
Other	Psoriasis, multiple sclerosis

* Adapted from Murray *et al.*, 1988.

to one selected antigen. Some of the diseases in which IFNγ deficiencies have been found are outlined in Table 9.3. Deficient IFNγ production is also involved in the ongoing IgE synthesis by B cells of atopic individuals. IgE production is IL-4-mediated and involves complex lymphokine interactions in which the IL-4-induced IgE responses are positively or negatively modulated. The antagonist role played by IFNγ in this system is crucial. Formation of IgE by CD4-positive helper cells is the net result of the enhancing and suppressing effects of IL-4 and IFNγ, respectively, both of which are secreted by T cells upon activation. In atopic individuals with elevated IgE levels, mononuclear cells produce high levels of IL-4 and low levels of IFNγ as compared to the mononuclear cells of healthy donors (Pane, 1989). It therefore seems that, in certain individuals, predominant IL-4 production will support IgE antibody response, whereas, in other individuals, IFNγ will be predominantly produced and thus drive the antibody response to other isotypes.

IFNγ antagonists The use of soluble IFNγ receptor and monoclonal antibodies to IFNγ may attenuate the processes outlined above (Garotta *et al.*, 1989). One of the most potent synthetic inhibitors of IFNγ mRNA production has been cyclosporin A. Other inhibitors include corticosteroids, prostaglandins, 1,25-dihydroxyvitamin D3, histamine and opioids such as β-endorphin (Young and Hardy, 1990).

INTERFERON-GAMMA IN THE CLINIC

Cancer

A significant number of phase I–II trials have assessed the efficacy and toxicity of IFNγ administered intravenously, intramuscularly and intraperitoneally. A lower maximum tolerated dose for 24 h (0.2-0.5×10^6 U/m^2) as compared to 6 h (3.2×10^6 U/m^2) and bolus (about 30×10^6 U/m^2) injections has been described (Kurzrock et al., 1986a,d; 1985; Brown et al. 1987). The maximum tolerated dose of intramuscular injections is intermediate (5-10×10^6 U/m^2) (Kurzrock et al., 1986a). Dose-limiting side-effects usually include high fever and fatigue.

Unfortunately, the vast majority of studies have not shown significant antitumour effects after administration of IFNγ, especially in patients with solid tumours. For example, Ernstoff, et al. (1987) treated 30 patients with metastatic melanoma with IFNγ by 2- or 24-h i.v. infusion for 14 days at doses ranging from 3 to 3000 mcg/m^2. There were two responses (a CR and PR) at the 3 mcg/m^2/day and 300 mcg/m^2/day dose levels respectively. Boman et al. (1988) performed a phase I study of IFNγ. Two responses were noted in 35 patients. D'Acquisto et al. (1988) failed to detect any responses in 27 patients with refractory ovarian cancer treated with intraperitoneal IFNγ. In this study, subjects experienced occasional fevers, mild myelosuppression and transient increases in hepatic transaminase, but no one was removed because of toxicity. Serum levels of IFNγ were detectable at doses $> 0.05 \times 10^6$ U/m^2 and reached 15 U/ml at the highest dose. There was a great pharmacologic advantage in that levels of up to 1720 U/ml were found in the peritoneal fluid. No responses were noted in phase II evaluations of IFNγ in patients with pancreatic carcinoma, renal carcinoma, or melanoma (Von Hoff et al., 1990; Creagan et al., 1990) Similarly, in our phase I–II studies, which included over 100 patients, few responses were seen (Kurzrock et al., 1985; 1986a, d; Quesada et al., 1988).

Some responses have been noted in haematological disorders. In one study of myelodysplastic syndrome, 60% of patients treated with 0.1 mg/m^2/day of IFNγ showed improvement in haematological parameters and perhaps a survival advantage (Maiolo et al., 1990); confirmation of this observation by other investigators has not yet been published. A study by our group has shown that IFNγ can induce haematological remission and cytogenetic responses in a small proportion (20-25%) of patients with CML (Kurzrock et al., 1987). IFNγ is not effective in many of the B-cell diseases which are responsive to IFNα, e.g. hairy-cell leukaemia, multiple myeloma (Quesada et al., 1988).

IFNγ has shown in vitro synergy with IFNα and tumour necrosis factor-alpha (TNFα). However, combining these cytokines in the clinic has proved problematic. For instance, in the case of IFNγ and IFNα combinations, synergistic toxicity was observed, with the maximum tolerated dose of the combination being 2×10^6 U/m^2/day total interferon dose (1×10^6 U/m^2/day of each interferon) (Kurzrock et al., 1986c). In contrast, the maximum tolerated dose of either IFNγ or IFNα administered alone is 5×10^6 U/m^2/day. Further, in a phase II study of patients with CML, in which we gave combined IFNγ and IFNα therapy, either concomitantly or sequentially, the results were not improved over those obtained after administration of IFNα alone (R Kurzrock and M Talpaz, unpublished data). A lowering of the maximum tolerated dose was also observed when IFNγ was combined with TNFα (Kurzrock et al., 1988).

Chronic granulomatous disease

Chronic granulomatous disease (CGD) is an hereditary disorder characterized by recurrent pyogenic infections. Phagocytes from patients with this disease are able to ingest, but not to kill, certain organisms due to failure of cellular NADPH oxidase to produce superoxide. In normal cells, IFNγ substantially increases the level of transcripts for the enzyme – IFNα decreases the level of transcription (Newburger et al., 1988). IFNγ has been tested in patients with CGD and has been found to partially correct the defect in superoxide production and the very low level of cytochrome b heavy-chain gene expression. These salutary effects may be sufficient to allow restoration of monocyte and granulocyte antimicrobial functions, as demonstrated by significant improvement in phagocyte bactericidal activity against Staphylococcus aureus.

The observations in CGD provide a model for the pharmacological modulation of gene expression and the use of interferons as an adjunct to more conventional aproaches to the management of microbial, and, perhaps, neoplastic diseases.

IgE production

IFNγ inhibits the IL-4-induced synthesis of IgE by peripheral blood mononuclear cells. Peripheral blood mononuclear cells from children with hyper-IgE syndrome produce lower concentrations of IFNγ than mononuclear cells from healthy controls. Analysis at the clonal level reveals that patients with hyper IgE syndrome have significantly lower proportions of circulating

T cells that can produce IFNγ and TNFα, but not of T cells producing IL-2 or IL-4, in comparison with controls.

A recent report on patients with Job's Syndrome (an immunodeficiency characterized by high serum concentrations of IgE, chronic eczema and recurrent bacterial infections) has shown significant decreases in IgE values after subcutaneous injection of IFNγ (King *et al.*, 1989). IFNγ has also demonstrated clinical efficacy in the treatment of atopic dermatitis associated with high IgE production (Boguniewicz *et al.*, 1990).

Non-viral infections

Harms and co-workers (1989) treated patients with cutaneous leishmaniasis with intradermal injections of 20-25 mcg of IFNγ on four occasions, 2 days apart. Responses were seen in patients who had *Leishmania braziliensis guyanensis* and in those who had *L. tropica,* though the responses were more pronounced in the latter group. Indeed, 9 of 13 *L. tropica* lesions resolved completely within 4–8 weeks. There were no local or systemic adverse reactions. Immunohistochemical studies suggested that the responses may have been due to enhanced cell-mediated immunity.

IFNγ has also induced partial to marked responses in a small number of patients with lepromatous leprosy, AIDS-related *M. avium-intracellulare* and tranfusion-acquired Chaga's disease (Murray, 1990).

Hepatitis and other disorders

A trial of combined IFNγ and IFNβ has shown efficacy in chronic active hepatitis B (Caselmann *et al.*, 1989) with five of ten patients showing a response. However, in a randomized study of IFNα versus IFNγ in hepatitis C, only the patients treated with IFNα responded (Saez-Royuela *et al.*, 1991).

In a randomized trial, administration of low-dose (50 mcg/day) subcutaneous IFNγ resulted in significant and prolonged improvement in patients with rheumatoid arthritis (Lemmel *et al.*, 1988). However, in another study, a statistically significant difference was not seen (Cannon *et al.*, 1989). There are also anecdotal reports of improvement in patients with systematic sclerosis. Administration of IFNγ to patients with multiple sclerosis has been associated with exacerbation of disease (Johnson, 1988).

INTERFERON-GAMMA

CONCLUSION

IFNγ is a cytokine derived predominantly from T cells and NK cells. It is structurally and functionally distinct from the other interferons. Antiviral, antiproliferative and antimicrobial effects are included amongst its protean biological activities. However, it is most potent as an immunomodulator. Indeed, it can alter most immune functions. In addition to human peripheral blood monocytes and monocyte-derived macrophages, the spectrum of host defence cells capable of responding to IFNγ with in vitro antimicrobial activity has been expanded to include human alveolar macrophages, human placental and peritoneal macrophages and murine hepatic macrophages (Kupffer cells). Although not usually considered to be host defence cells in the traditional sense of the phagocytic leucocyte, human and murine fibroblasts, human endothelial, epithelial and parenchymal cells, and astrocytes have also been shown to respond to IFNγ with intracellular microbicidal or microbistatic activity.

In spite of its broad range of in vitro immune activity, a large number of clinical trials have failed to show efficacy for IFNγ as an antitumour agent. Modulation of gene function in chronic granulomatous disease and in states with high IgE levels, and improvement in infections in some non-viral disorders may prove to be novel applications for this molecule. As over-production of IFNγ has been associated with certain inflammatory and autoimmune disorders, investigations of the therapeutic role for IFNγ antagonists, i.e. soluble receptors, monoclonal antibodies, and small molecules that interfere with ligand/receptor interaction, is warranted.

REFERENCES

Boguniewicz M, Jaffe HS, Izu A et al. (1990). Recombinant gamma interferon in treatment of patients with atopic dermatitis and elevated IgE levels. Am J Med. **88**, 365–70.

Bonnem EM, Oldham RK (1987). Gamma Interferon: Physiology and potential role in cancer therapy. J Biol Response Mod. **6**, 275–301.

Boman BM, Gagen MM and Bonnem et al. (1988). Phase I study of recombinant gamma interferon. J Biol Response Mod. **7**, 438–42.

Branca AA, Faltynek CR, D'Allessandro SB and Baglioni C (1982). Interaction of interferon with cellular receptors, internalisation and degradation of cell-bound interferon. J Biol Chem. **257**, 13291–6.

Brown TD, Koeller J, Beogher K et al. (1987). A phase I clinical trial of recombinant DNA gamma interferon. J Clin Oncol. **5**, 790–8.

R. KURZROCK

Cannon GW, Pincus SH, Emkey RD *et al.* (1989). Double-blind trial of recombinant γ-interferon versus placebo in the treatment of rheumatoid arthritis. *Arthritis Rheum.* **8**, 964–73.

Capobianchi MR, Ameglio F, Tosi R and Dolei A (1985). Differences in the expression and release of DR, BR, and DQ molecules in human cells treated with recombinant interferon gamma: comparison to other interferons. *Hum Immunol.* **13**, 1–11.

Caselmann WH, Eisenburg J, Hofschneider PH and Koshy R (1989). β- and γ– interferon in chronic active hepatitis B: A pilot trial of short-term combination therapy. *Gastroenterology.* **96**, 449–55.

Creagan ET, Schaid DJ, Ahmann DL and Frytak S (1990). Disseminated malignant melanoma and recombinant inteferon: Analysis of seven consecutive Phase II investigations. *J Invest Dermatol.* **95**, 188S–192S.

D'Acquisto R, Markman M, Hakes T *et al.* (1988). A Phase I trial of intraperitoneal recombinant gamma interferon in advanced ovarian carcinoma. *J Clin Oncol.* **6**, 689–74.

Dianzoni F and Baron S (1975). Unexpectedly rapid action of human interferon in physiological conditions. *Nature.* **257**, 682–4.

Ernstoff MS, Trautman T, Davis CA *et al.* (1987). A randomised Phase I/II study of continuous versus intermittent intravenous interferon in patients with metastatic melanoma. *J Clin Oncol.* **4**, 1804–8.

Garotta G, Ozmen L and Fountoulakis M (1989). Development of IFN-γ antagonists as an example of biotechnology application to approach new immunomodulators. *Pharmacol Res.* **21 (Suppl. 2)**, 5–17.

Giedlund MA, Orn H, Wigzell H, Senik A and Gresser I (1987). Enhanced NK cell activity in mice injected with interferon and interferon inducers. *Nature.* **273**, 759–63.

Gutterman JU, Rosenblum MG, Rios AA *et al.* (1984). Pharamcokinetic study of partially pure gamma-interferon in cancer patients. *Cancer Res.* **44**, 4164–71.

Handa K, Suzuki R, Matsui H *et al.* (1983). Natural killer (NK) cells as a responder to interleukin 2 (IL 2). II. IL 2-induced IFN-gamma production. *J. Immunol.* **130**, 988–92.

Harms G, Zwingenberger K and Chehade AK *et al.* (1989). Effects of intradermal gamma-interferon in cutaneous leishmaniasis..*Lancet* .**8650**, 1287–92.

Ijzermans JNM and Marquet RL (1989). IFN-gamma: A review. *Immunobiology.* **179**, 456–73.

Johnson KP (1988). Treatment of multiple sclerosis with various interferons: The cons. *Neurology.* **38**, 62–5.

Jurado A, Carballido J, Griffel H *et al.* (1989). The immunomodulatory effects of IFN-gamma on mature B-lymphocyte responses. *Experientia.* **45**, 521–6.

Kasahara T, Hooks JJ, Dougherty SF and Oppenheim JJ (1983). Interleukin 2-mediated immune interferon (IFN-γ) production by human T cells and T cell subsets. *J Immunol.* **130**, 1784–9.

King CL, Gallin JI, Maelch HL *et al.* (1989). Regulation of immunoglobulin production in hyperimmunoglobulin and recurrent infection syndrome by interferon gamma. *Proc Natl Acad Sci USA.* **86**, 1085–9.

Kleinerman ES, Kurzrock R, Wyatt D *et al.* (1986). Activation or suppression of the tumoricidal properties of monocytes from cancer patients following treatment with human recombinant gamma-interferon. *Cancer Res.* **46**, 5401–5.

Kurzrock R, Rosenblum MG, Sherwin SA *et al.* (1985). Pharmacokinetics, single-dose tolerance, and biological activity of recombinant gamma-interferon in cancer patients. *Cancer Res.* **45** 2866–72.

Kurzrock R, Quesada JR, Talpaz M *et al.* (1986a). Phase I study of multiple dose intramuscularly administered recombinant gamma interferon. *J Clin Oncol.* **4**, 1101–9.

Kurzrock R, Rohde MF, Quesada JR *et al.* (1986b). Recombinant gamma interferon induces hypertriglyceridemia and inhibits post-heparin lipase activity in cancer patients. *J Exp Med.* **164**, 1093–101.

Kurzrock R, Rosenblum MG, Quesada JR *et al.* (1986c). Phase I study of a combination of recombinant IFN-alpha and recombinant IFN-gamma in cancer patients. *J Clin Oncol.* **4**, 1677–83.

Kurzrock R, Quesada JR, Rosenblum MG *et al.* (1986d). Phase I study of IV administered recombinant gamma interferon in cancer patients. *Cancer Treat Rep.* **70**, 1357–64.

Kurzrock R, Talpaz M, Kantarjian H *et al.* (1987). Therapy of chronic myelogenous leukaemia with recombinant interferon-gamma. *Blood.* **70**, 943–7.

Kurzrock R, Feinberg B, Talpaz M, Saks S and Gutterman JU (1988). Phase I study of a combination of recombinant tumour necrosis factor-α and recombinant interferon-gamma in cancer patients. *J Interferon Res.* **9**, 435–44.

Kurzrock R, Talpaz M and Gutterman JU (1991). Interferons-α, β, γ: Basic principles and preclinical studies. In: *Biologic Therapy of Cancer;* ed. Devita VT, Hellman S, Rosenberg SA, Philadelphia: Lippincott Co, Inc. 247–74.

Le J, Lin JX, Henriksen-Destafano D and Vilcek J (1986). Bacterial lipooplysaccharide-induced IFN-gamma production: roles of interleukin 1 and interleukin 2. *J Immunol.* **135**, 4525–30.

Lemmel E-M, Obert HJ and Hofschneider PH (1988). Low dose gamma interferon in treatment of rheumatoid arthritis. *Lancet.* **1**, 595–8.

Maiolo AT, Cortelezzi A, Calori R and Polli EE (1990). Recombinant γ-interferon as first line therapy for high risk myelodysplastic syndromes. *Leukaemia.* **4**, 480–5.

Maluish AE, Urba WJ, Gordon K *et al.* (1987). Determination of an optimum biological response modifying (BRM) dose of interferon gamma in melanoma patients (Abstract). *Proc Am Soc Clin Oncol.* **6**, 251.

Murray HW (1988). IFN-gamma, the activated macrophage, and host defence against microbial challenge. *Ann Intern Med.* **108**, 595–608.

Murray HW (1990). Gamma interferon, cytokine-induced macrophage activation, and anti-microbial host defense. *Diagn Microbiol Infect Dis.* **13**, 411–21.

Murray JL, Stuckey SE, Pillow JK *et al.* (1988). Differential in vitro effects of recombinant α-interferon and recombinant gamma-interferon alone or in combination on the expression of melanoma-associated surface antigens. *J Biol Resonse Mod.* **7**, 152–61.

Nakagawara A, Desantis NM, Nogueira N and Nathan CG (1982). Lymphokines enhance the capacity of human monocytes to secrete reactive oxygen intermediates. *J Clin Invest.* **70**, 1042–51.

Nathan C (1986). IFN-gamma and macrophage activation in cell-mediated immunity. In: Mechanisms of host resistance to infectious agents, tumours and allografts; ed. Stenman RM. Norht RJ. New York: Rockefeller University Press. 165–84.

Newburger PE, Ezekowitz AB, Whitney C, Wright J and Orkin SH (1988). Induction of phagocyte cytochrome b heavy chain gene expression by IFN-gamma. *Proc Natl Acad Sci USA.* **85**, 5215–19.

Nugent KM, Glazier J, Monick MM and Hunninghake GW (1985). Stimulated human alveolar macrophages secrete interferon. *Am Rev Respir Dis.* **131**, 714–18.

Pane J (1989). Regulatory role of cytokines and CD23 in the human IgE antibody synthesis. *Int Arch Allergy Appl Immunol.* **90**, 32–40.

Queseda DR, Alexanaian R, Kurzrock R *et al.* (1988). Recombinant interferon gamma in hairy cell leukaemia, multiple myeloma, and Waldenstrom's macroglobulinemia. *Am J Hematol.* **29**, 1–4.

Rubin BY and Gupta SL (1980). Differential efficacies of human type I and type II interferons as antiviral and antiproliferative agents. *Proc Natl Acad Sci USA.* **77**, 5928–32.

Saez-Royuela F, Porres JC, Moreno A *et al.* (1991). High doses of recombinant α-interferon or γ-interferon for chronic hepatitis C: randomised, controlled trial. *Hepatology.* **13**, 327–31.

Shalaby MR, Hamilton EB, Benninger AH and Marafino BJ (1985). In vivo antiviral activity of recombinant murine gamma interferon. *J Interferon Res.* **5**, 339–45.

Sidman CL, Marshall JD, Shultz LD, Gray PW and Johnson HM (1984). Gamma-interferon is one of several direct B cell-maturing lymphokines. *Nature.* **309**, 801–4.

Thompson JA, Cox WW, Lindgren CG *et al.* (1987). Subcutaneous recombinant gamma interferon in cancer patients: toxicity, pharmacokinetics, and immunomodulatory effects. *Cancer Immunol Immunother.* **25**, 47–53.

Torok-Storb B, Johnson GG, Bowden R and Storb R (1987). Gamma-interferon in aplastic anaemia: Inability to detect significant levels in sera or demonstrate haematopoietic suppressing activity. *Blood.* **72**, 629–33.

Ucer U, Bartsch H, Scheurich P and Pfizenmaier K (1985). Biological effects of gamma interferon on human tumour cells; quantity and affinity of cell membrane receptors for gamma interferon in relation to growth inhibition and induction of HLA-DR expression. *Int J Cancer.* **36**, 103–8.

Van der Burg M, Edelstein M, Gerlis L *et al.* (1985). Recombinant IFN-gamma (Immuneron): Results of a phase I trial in patients with cancer. *J Biol Response Mod.* **4**, 264–72.

Von Hoff DD, Fleming TR, MacDonald JS *et al.* (1990). Phase II evaluation of recombinant γ-interferon in patients with advanced pancreatic carcinoma: A Southwest oncology group study. *J Biol Response Mod.* **9**, 584–7.

Wagstaff J, Smith D, Nelmes P, Loynds P and Crowther D (1987). A phase I study of recombinant interferon gamma administered by s.c. injection three times per week in patients with solid tumours. *Cancer Immunol Immunother.* **25**, 54–8.

Welsh RM, Yang H and Bukowski JF (1988). The role of interferon in the regulation of virus infections by cytotoxic lymphocytes. *Bioessays.* **8**, 10–13.

Young HA and Hardy KJ (1990). IFN-γ Producer cells, activation stimuli and molecular genetic regulation. *Pharmacol Ther.* **45**, 137–51.

Zoon KC (1987). Human Interferons: Structure and function. In: Interferon 9; ed. I Gresser, 1–12. London: Academic Press.

Zoumbos NC, Gascon P, Djeu JY and Young NS (1985). Interferon is a mediator of haematopoietic suppression in aplastic anaemia in vitro and possibly in vivo. *Proc Natl Acad Sci USA.* **82**, 188–92.

10

TUMOUR NECROSIS FACTOR

A. A. REGE, K. HUANG and B. B. AGGARWAL

INTRODUCTION

Tumour necrosis factor (TNF) is one of the most pleiotropic and pluripotent cytokines known, and shares several overlapping and interacting properties with other members of the cytokine family (Aggarwal and Vilcek, 1991).

Originally defined as a factor produced in Bacille–Calmette–Guerin (BCG)-primed animals in response to endotoxin, TNF was named for its ability to necrotize a variety of tumours (O'Malley et al., 1962; Carswell et al., 1975). The designation 'alpha' (TNFα) was later added to distinguish it from a related cytokine, TNFβ, also known as lymphotoxin (LT). In this chapter we will refer to TNFα as TNF, and to TNFβ as LT. Cachectin, first described as a factor responsible for cachexia, was later shown to be identical to TNF (Beutler et al., 1985). Alternate names have been used in the literature to describe this protein, e.g. macrophage cytotoxin, necrosin, cytotoxin, hemorrhagic factor, macrophage cytotoxic factor and differentiation-inducing factor (Aggarwal, 1991a). Furthermore, based on its multiple functions, TNF has been categorized as a monokine, a lymphokine, a growth factor and a mitogen.

A variety of bioassays exploiting the cytotoxic effects of TNF on target cells have been developed (Aggarwal and Kohr, 1985). However, such assays do not distinguish between TNF and LT, and this has led to the development of specific immunoassays.

Treatment of animals with endotoxin has been shown to cause hyperplasia of macrophages, suggesting that these cells are the primary source of TNF (Carswell et al., 1975). Subsequently, a number of other cells were found to be capable of secreting TNF, including natural killer (NK) cells, astrocytes, lymphocytes, Kupffer cells, smooth muscle cells, keratinocytes, glial cells, neutrophils, granulosa cells, fibroblasts, endothelial cells and many tumour cells (Spriggs *et al.*, 1991).

TNF is rarely detected in the body fluids of healthy individuals, but has been found in human breast milk and normal amniotic fluid (Jaatella *et al.*, 1988; Mushtaha *et al.*, 1989). In various pathological states TNF has been detected in serum, cerebrospinal fluid, synovial fluid, bronchial lavage fluid, vesical fluid and lymph. Upon stimulation, serum TNF rapidly reaches high levels. However, it has a short half-life (5–25 min) and disappears very rapidly upon removal of the stimulus.

Commercial preparations of recombinant human TNF are now available from different manufacturers; although these agents vary slightly in their amino acid sequences they show no detectable differences in biological activity.

PHYSICOCHEMICAL PROPERTIES

TNF was first isolated and purified to homogeneity from the conditioned culture medium of a human promyelomonocytic cell line, HL-60 (Aggarwal *et al.*, 1985). Since then, the molecule has been purified from several sources (Aggarwal, 1991b), but as human TNF remains by far the most studied it is discussed here as the representative molecule.

Human TNF has a molecular mass of 17 kDa, as determined by SDS–PAGE and 45 kDa, as determined by gel filtration, suggesting that the native molecule is oligomeric. Natural human TNF exists as a non-glycosylated protein with an isoelectric point of approximately 5.3. The monomer is 157 amino acids long and contains two cysteines, forming an intramolecular disulphide bridge. Substantial interspecies homology indicates evolutionary conservation (Goeddel *et al.*, 1986). TNF also shows significant amino acid sequence similarity to LT (Aggarwal *et al.*, 1985b).

Molecular weight determination by ultracentrifugation suggests that the native molecule is a compact trimer (Arakawa and Yphantis, 1987). The oligomerization does not appear to be due to the formation of intermolecular disulphide bonds, but rather appears to be a result of non-covalent interactions (Davis *et al.*, 1987). Even though it is generally believed that the trimeric form of TNF is biologically active, monomeric and dimeric forms have also been isolated. Recent analysis of its tertiary structure by X-ray crystallography has confirmed that human TNF is a non-helical, trimeric molecule containing antiparallel ß sheets (Jones *et al.*, 1990). Further, it has

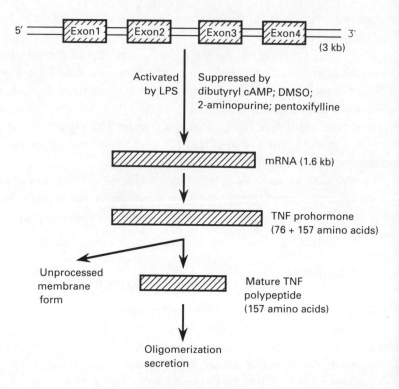

Fig. 10.1. Biosynthesis and processing of human TNF. DMSO, dimethyl sulphoxide; LPS, lipopolysaccharide.

been noted that the monomers are packed in a jelly-roll motif, resembling the structure of coat proteins of certain viruses, including foot and mouth necrosis virus and satellite tobacco necrosis virus. The significance of this similarity is not known.

Human TNF is synthesized as a prohormone containing 233 amino acids, whereas the mature polypeptide is 157 amino acids long (Pennica *et al.*, 1984). The propeptide portion is 76 amino acids long and must be processed proteolytically to generate the mature, secreted 17-kDa TNF (Fig. 10.1). Recently, a 26 kDa, transmembrane form of TNF was found and was shown to be active in cell-to-cell contact-mediated cytotoxicity (Kriegler *et al.,* 1988; Perez *et al.,* 1990). It also has been suggested that the transmembrane form may act as a receptor for soluble TNF receptor, which itself may have cytokine-like actions (Porteu and Nathan, 1990).

TUMOUR NECROSIS FACTOR

Gene structure and regulation

In man, the TNF gene is located on chromosome 6, in close proximity to the major histocompatibility complex (MHC) and LT genes (Spies *et al.*, 1989). Such close clustering of these genes is perhaps relevant in terms of their evolution and importance in the immune system. Molecular cloning has revealed that the coding region of the TNF gene is divided into four exons, arranged over approximately 3 kb of total DNA (Fig. 10.1). Considerable sequence conservation is found within the coding regions of the TNF genes of different species. In addition, there are highly conserved sequences in both the 5' and the 3' flanking (untranslated) regions, presumably associated with TNF gene regulation.

It is apparent that regulation of TNF biosynthesis occurs at multiple levels (Spriggs *et al.*, 1990). The cytokine is produced in a tissue-specific manner, with different cells exhibiting different levels of expression, either constitutively or in response to a variety of stimuli. Production is best understood in monocytes and macrophages. Unstimulated macrophages possess untranslated precursors of TNF that are translated to produce the mature molecule within minutes of exposure to bacterial lipopolysaccharide (LPS) (Beutler *et al.*, 1986). A variety of inducing stimuli has been described – viruses, bacteria, fungi, tumour cells, phorbol esters, cytokines (TNF, IL-1, GM-CSF, IFNs, IL-2), Fc receptor cross-linking and free oxygen radicals. Inhibitory stimuli include prostaglandin E2, cAMP, dexamethasone, IL-4, IL-6 and botulinum D toxin (Spriggs *et al.*, 1991). In most cases, the regulatory mechanism is not well understood, in either myeloid or non-myeloid cells.

Signal transduction

Receptors   The first step in the action of TNF is its binding to a high-affinity cell surface receptor. Both the secreted and the membrane-anchored forms of this ligand can bind to the receptor, leading to an unusually diverse array of cellular responses (Kronke *et al.*, 1991). The versatility in TNF action can be partly attributed to the fact that its receptors are present on virtually all cells examined, yet exhibit structural and functional heterogeneity. In addition, binding results in the activation of several signal transduction pathways and the induction of an unusually large array of cellular genes.

Recently, two distinct TNF receptors, with molecular weights of 55–60 kDa and 75–85 kDa, also referred to as p60 (TNF-RI or TNF-R-a) and p80 (TNF-RII or TNF-R-b), respectively, have been identified and their cDNAs cloned (Gray *et al.*, 1990; Sprang, 1990). The extracellular portions of the two receptors exhibit 28% amino acid sequence homology to each other and also to that of the nerve growth factor receptor, together forming a receptor family. In contrast, no significant similarity is found between the intracytoplasmic portions of the two TNF receptors, suggesting that the two receptors may activate different intracellular signalling pathways (Dembic *et al*, 1990).

Most cell lines examined have both receptors, expressed in different proportions; however, some cell lines express only the p60 receptor (Dembic *et al.*, 1990), suggesting that one receptor type is perhaps sufficient for high-affinity binding and full biological activity.

Signal transduction pathways   Neither TNF nor its receptors possess intrinsic protein kinase activity. After binding to its specific receptor, TNF is internalized in clathrin-coated vesicles, moves to endosomes and to multilamellar bodies, and finally ends up in the lysosomes, where it is broken down (Mosselmans *et al.*, 1988). It has been suggested that TNF receptors perhaps function as transmembrane transporters for TNF, which upon internalization may serve as the intracellular signal; this process is known as endocytosis-mediated transduction (Yoshimura *et al.*, 1990). It recently has been demonstrated that TNF kills L929 fibroblasts when microinjected directly into the cells, suggesting that internalization may have a role in signal transduction (Smith *et al.*, 1990).

To date, no single universal second messenger for TNF signal transduction has been identified, but a significant body of evidence suggests that several messenger systems are activated in different systems (Fig. 10.2) (Kronke *et al.*, 1991). Thus, effects of TNF such as killing of L929 cells and inhibition of lipoprotein lipase activity in 3T3L1 adipocytes have been shown to be reversed by pertussis toxin, suggesting that G proteins are involved in signalling (Earl *et al.*, 1990). In human fibroblasts, it has been demonstrated that there is an increase in adenylate cyclase activity, leading to an accumulation of cAMP and an increase in protein kinase A (PKA) activity (Zhang *et al.*, 1988). The cytokine may be activating adenylate cyclase via G proteins or via protein kinase C (PKC). Agents that increase intracellular cAMP, such as prostaglandin E, are synergistic with TNF (Scholz and Altman, 1989). Activation of PKC by several pathways has been demonstrated in several cell lines (Schutze *et al.*, 1990). These activated protein kinases are responsible for the phosphorylation of a number of cellular proteins that presumably channel TNF signals, e.g. stress/heat shock proteins, an mRNA cap-binding protein, epidermal growth factor receptor (Marino *et al.*, 1991).

Another set of reactions prominent in TNF signal transduction is the activation of phospholipases. Phospholipase A2 (PLA2), a G protein coupled

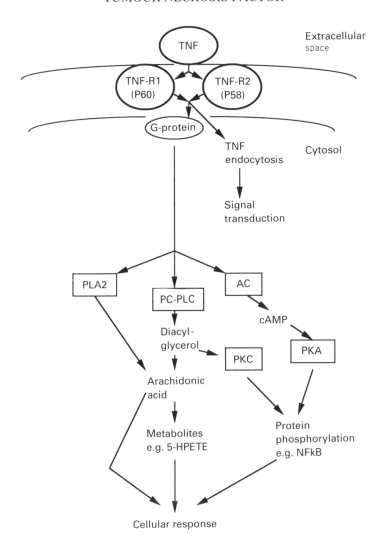

Fig. 10.2. TNF-induced signal transduction pathways. PLA2, phospholipase A2; PC-PLC, phosphatidylcholine-specific phospholipase C; AC, adenylate cyclase; PKA, protein kinase A; PKC, protein kinase C.

enzyme, has been shown to be activated in murine L-929S tumour cells during their in vitro killing by this cytotoxin (Knauer et al., 1990). Phospholipase C does not appear to be activated. However, a phosphatidylcholine-specific phospholipase C (PC-PLC) appears to be activated, resulting in the production of diacylglycerol (DAG), a potent activator of PKC and also a precursor of arachidonic acid. Phospholipase activation has been demonstrated in both TNF-mediated growth stimulation and inhibition (Palombella and Vilcek, 1989). TNF induction does not appear to involve an increase in either intracellular calcium or inositol phosphate (Spriggs *et al.*, 1990).

The action of either PLA2 or DAG lipase can result in the production of arachidonic acid, a key intermediate event in TNF signal transduction (Neale *et al.*, 1988). Arachidonic acid itself or its metabolites, such as 5-HPETE (Haliday *et al.*, 1991), may act as second messengers.

Effect on cellular genes   Early studies showed that inhibitors of protein (e.g. cycloheximide) and RNA (actinomycin D) synthesis greatly increase the cytotoxicity of TNF. Recently, it has been shown that a number of genes are either switched on or switched off by TNF and may be involved in the pleiotropic actions of this cytokine (Kronke *et al.*, 1991). Activated genes include those for several cytokines and growth factors, receptors, cell adhesion molecules, inflammatory mediators, acute-phase proteins, MHC proteins, retroviral proteins, numerous transcription (and a few translation) factors and other miscellaneous proteins. Nuclear transcription factors are of particular interest because they act as substrates for activated protein kinases and serve as third messengers. Examples of transcription factors induced by TNF include NFkB, AP-1, IRF-1 and NF-GMa.

Recently, it was shown in several cell types that initiation of mRNA translation is regulated by TNF via the phosphorylation of an mRNA cap binding protein (eukaryotic initiation factor 4E) involved in selecting specific messages for translation (Marino *et al.*, 1991). TNF also inhibits several cellular genes, e.g. *c-myc*, collagen, and thrombomodulin, the target cell type determining whether a particular gene is activated or suppressed.

BIOLOGICAL EFFECTS OF TNF

Over the years, a bewildering variety of biological effects have been elucidated using both in vitro and in vivo systems: these will now be discussed.

In vitro effects

The various effects of this cytokine have been measured in terms of cell proliferation, DNA synthesis and induction of products such as prostaglandins, collagen, HLA, stromelysin, cytokines (including TNF itself), growth factors and transcription factors. Many of these observations are teleologically consistent with the involvement of TNF in numerous pathophysiological processes, e.g. inflammation, immunity, tumorigenesis. Highlighted below are the best-known examples of cellular effects of TNF, classified according to major cell types.

Tumour cells Lines susceptible to the effects of TNF include carcinoma, sarcoma, glioma and melanoma, some of which are resistant to anticancer drugs (Salmon *et al.*, 1985). Such inhibitory effects can be enhanced by the simultaneous use of other agents, e.g. IFNγ, IL-1 and IL-2 and retinoic acid. Conversely, TNF stimulates certain tumour cell lines (e.g. human cervical carcinoma, astrocytoma and osteosarcoma cells). However, the majority of cell lines (untransformed included) are resistant to TNF-mediated killing (Vilcek and Palombella, 1991).

Whether the ultimate effect on the target cell is stimulatory or inhibitory depends on factors such as ligand concentration, presence of protein and RNA synthesis inhibitors, and presence of other cytokines. The mechanism of the antiproliferative effects of TNF is not well understood. Some of the reported effects on target cells include DNA fragmentation, alteration in arachidonic acid metabolism, lipid peroxidation and involvement of lysosomal enzymes such as proteases. However, it has not been possible to correlate any single cellular or biochemical characteristic (e.g. presence of oncogenes, receptor concentration, cellular lineage) with sensitivity to TNF. Anaerobic conditions, antioxidants, corticosteroids and superoxide dismutases are known to block the deleterious effects of this cytotoxin (Wong *et al*, 1989).

Haematopoietic and lymphoid cells The versatility of TNF is apparent when one considers that the agent can affect primitive, differentiated and neoplastic cells. Thus, upon TNF exposure, colony formation and proliferation of erythroid progenitor cells are suppressed, whereas differentiation and proliferation of myelomonocytic cells are enhanced (Broxmeyer *et al.*, 1986; Roodman *et al*, 1987). The monokine has also been shown to be chemotactic for blood monocytes and neutrophils (Ming *et al.*, 1987). A complex array of responses is displayed by neutrophils, including increased degranulation (Klebanoff *et al*, 1986), phagocytosis and antibody-dependent cellular cytotoxicity (Shalaby *et al.*, 1985), enhanced production of reactive oxygen radicals (Nathan, 1987) and CD11b/CD18 adhesion molecules (Gamble *et al.*, 1985). Macrophages respond to TNF by down-regulating certain oncogenes and by increasing the production of prostaglandins and cytokines, including MCSF-1, GM-CSF, IL-1, IL-6 and IL-8 (Matsushima *et al*, 1988) and even TNF itself (autocrine regulation).

Mitogenic effects of TNF are seen with T and B cells (Andrews *et al.*, 1990). In mature human T cells, induction of IFNγ, IL-2 receptor and MHC I

A. A. REGE, K. HUANG & B. B. AGGARWAL

has been observed. Eosinophils produce oxidants, increasing their toxicity towards human endothelium (Slungaard *et al.*, 1990).

Endothelial and muscle cells TNF modulates antigen expression, cell morphology, viability, and adhesive properties of endothelial cells (Beutler and Cerami, 1988). The resultant metabolic changes have been taken as evidence that this growth modulator plays an important role in such unrelated physiological processes as angiogenesis and capillary leak syndrome. These various effects are seen as induction by these cells of IL-1, GM-CSF, ICAM-1, HLA and tissue factor but suppression of activated protein C and thrombomodulin expression. It has been shown recently that TNF and IFNγ synergistically induce mouse brain microvascular cells in vitro to produce nitric oxide, a substance known to cause hypotension in vivo (Kilbourn and Belloni, 1990). Skeletal muscle fibres have been shown to experience a TNF-induced decrease in the resting transmembrane potential difference, leading to perturbation of membrane function (Tracey *et al*, 1986).

Connective and skeletal tissue effects Upon exposure to TNF, growth of several lines of normal human fibroblasts is enhanced (Sugarman *et al.*, 1985), prompting the use of the term 'growth factor' in describing TNF (Vilcek and Palombella, 1991). TNF induces osteoblastic cells to stimulate osteoclastic bone resorption and inhibits new bone formation (Mundy *et al.*, 1991). In cultured rat calvariae, the cytokine is mitogenic, leading to an increased number of collagen-synthesizing cells; however, it also has a direct inhibitory effect on osteoblastic function (Canalis, 1987). In chondrocytes, DNA and collagenase synthesis are induced, cartilage turnover is increased and glycosaminoglycan synthesis is suppressed (Ikebe *et al.*, 1988).

Other cell types TNF causes enhancement of several acute-phase reactants in hepatoma cell lines, including the complement proteins factor B and factor C3 and A-1 antichymotrypsin; at the same time, it induces suppression of albumin and transferrin (Perlmutter *et al.*, 1986). Adipocytes show enhanced lipolysis and suppressed biosynthesis of lipoprotein lipase and fatty acid synthetase in response to TNF (reviewed in Beutler and Cerami, 1988). The pro-inflammatory capacity of kidney mesangial cells is also modulated by TNF by induction of oxygen radical production (Radeke *et al.*, 1990). The cytokine induces prostaglandin production in human amnion cells and is cytostatic to these cells (Casey *et al.*, 1989). TNF causes demyelination and death of oligodendrocytes, suggesting a role in neurological disease (Selman and Raine, 1988).

160

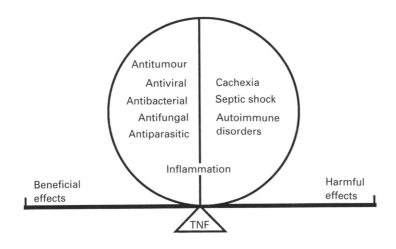

Fig. 10.3. The beneficial and harmful effects of human TNF.

In vivo effects

TNF has both beneficial and harmful effects, depending on the concentration of TNF and the presence of other mediators (Fig. 10.3). TNF has now been firmly established as a 'cytokine' relevant to neoplasia, infectious disease, inflammation, immunity, tissue repair and remodelling, and angiogenesis. Perhaps the single most important physiological function one can attribute to this versatile molecule is a role in homeostasis (Tovey, 1988).

Antitumour activity The earliest significant discovery related to TNF was that the haemorrhagic necrosis of certain tumours is mediated by TNF induced as a result of certain bacterial infections. This and subsequent studies led to the ongoing interest in the potential clinical value of TNF as an antitumour agent (Balkwill, 1989). Its antitumour activity can be attributed to its effects on tumour vasculature, modulation of the immune system, and direct inhibition of tumour cell growth. The haemorrhage occurs selectively in the tumour and not in normal tissue, suggesting a difference between the vasculatures of the two tissues.

In recent years, the availability of rhTNF has greatly aided in establishing its activities, setting the stage for clinical trials. In vivo antitumour activity has been demonstrated against syngeneic murine tumours, human tumour xenografts in nude mice and fresh human tumours implanted in immunologically intact mice. Susceptibility of tumours to TNF appears to depend on factors such as the degree of vascularization and immunogenicity of the tumour cells.

TNF toxicity was a major problem in some studies and tended to vary from laboratory to laboratory. The presence of a subclinical infection, a problem not uncommon in laboratory mice, probably contributed to toxicity. Injecting rats with indomethacin or ibuprofen (both cyclo-oxygenase inhibitors), before TNF was administered, protected them against the toxic effects of the cytokine, suggesting that such a combination may have value to human patients (Kettelhut *et al.,* 1987; Marquet *et al.,* 1987).

Role in infectious disease The link between bacterial infections, tumour necrosis, and TNF was discussed earlier. In addition, certain bacterial infections result in 'septic shock syndrome', which is also mediated by TNF (discussed separately).

TNF also has been shown to be toxic to several infectious agents, either through its direct action or through its immunomodulatory effects. Thus, during murine infections caused by *Listeria monocytogenes* (Havell, 1987) and BCG (Kindler *et al.*, 1989), this monokine has been shown to activate macrophages and induce granuloma formation through an autoamplification process, ultimately resulting in the inhibition of these pathogens. Inhibitory effects also are seen against *Chlamydia* spp. (Shemer-Avni *et al.,* 1988), and DNA and RNA viruses (Wong and Goeddel, 1986).

In vitro treatment of cells with TNF, in combination with IFNγ, has been shown to reduce their susceptibility to the human immunodeficiency virus (HIV). Furthermore, this treatment is cytotoxic for HIV-infected cells (Wong *et al.*, 1988). However, use of TNF in the treatment of acquired immunodeficiency syndrome (AIDS)-related Kaposi's sarcoma has been unsuccessful in at least one clinical study (Aboulafie *et al.* 1989).

TNF can have both harmful and beneficial effects during parasitic infections. Thus, in African trypanosomiasis and cerebral malaria, it is the chief mediator of cachexia (discussed separately, see below). In contrast, it appears to play a protective role in infections caused by parasites such as *Leishmania major* (Titus *et al.,* 1989), *Schistosoma mansoni* (Damonneville *et al.*, 1988), *Trypanosoma cruzi* (Wirth and Kirszenbaum, 1988), *Plasmodium* spp. (Taverne *et al.*, 1987) and *Candida albicans* (Djeu *et al.*, 1986).

Inflammatory, haemorrhagic and related effects TNF is an endogenous pyrogen, and induces increased production of IL-1 (Dinarello *et al.*, 1986). The potent in vitro effects of TNF on neutrophils, monocytes, mast cells, fibroblasts and endothelial cells can account for its involvement in inflammation and haemorrhagic necrosis of tumours. In vivo evidence has been obtained by injection of TNF-inducing LPS, which produces 'acute phase' inflammation with neutrophil infiltration (Remick et al., 1990). TNF also is a chief mediator of the acute Shwartzman reaction induced by endotoxin (to be discussed later, see below).

Because of its growth modulatory effects on fibroblasts and endothelial cells, this 'growth factor' has been implicated in wound healing and tissue remodelling (Kahaleh et al., 1988). For example, it stimulates endothelial cells to produce procoagulant factor (tissue factor III), which can initiate the clotting cascade. Also, in contrast with in vitro toxic effects on endothelial cells, TNF can contribute to in vivo angiogenesis.

Immunomodulatory effects TNF is one of the key mediators of the systemic 'acute phase' or 'primary immune' response. Although its in vivo immunological role is not fully understood, its in vitro effects on haematopoietic and lymphoid cells strongly indicate that this protein has a multifaceted involvement in the immune system. For instance, injection of TNF causes decreased red blood cell mass and a profound anaemia in mice, suggesting a role in the suppression of erythropoiesis (Johnson et al., 1989). Also, when combined with an antigen, it has an adjuvant effect on T cell-dependent antibody responses. The various effects can be harmful, as seen in septic shock, or beneficial, as in protection against pathogens. For example, TNF, either alone or synergistically with IL-1, can be radioprotective if given one day prior to otherwise lethal doses of radiation (Neta, 1990).

Neuroendocrine effects TNF does not cross the blood–brain barrier. However, by affecting the neuroendocrine system, it contributes to the immune system–mediated stress response. Administration of TNF, or of LPS, which induces the cytokine, activates the hypothalamus–pituitary–adrenal or 'stress' axis, perhaps through the induction of IL-1 (McCann et al., 1990). This results in the release of adrenocorticotropic hormone and, subsequently, in the production of glucocorticoids. The latter have profound effects on the immune system.

Role in pathophysiology

Cachexia Cachexia is the state of net catabolism of stored protein and fat frequently associated with chronic disease such as parasitic infections and cancer. The syndrome also involves anaemia, mediated by disturbances in overall red blood cell metabolism. Cachexia can result from even a relatively low burden of a pathogen, indicating that the malnutrition is not caused by 'parasitic' nutrient depletion. Instead, it has been shown to be the end result of relatively high concentrations of host-derived cachectin/TNF, induced during certain diseases (Tracey and Cerami, 1991).

Injecting laboratory rats intraperitoneally with TNF has been shown to produce cachexia, complete with anorexia and weight loss. The pattern of weight loss in cachectic rats is different from that in partially starved rats. Thus, whereas the latter group loses only lipid, the cachectic rats lose both lipid and protein. Anti-TNF antibodies partially abrogate the development of anorexia and weight loss, thus suggesting a role for the cytokine in these symptoms of cachexia. Interestingly, upon long-term administration of TNF, cachectic rats develop tolerence (tachyphylaxis) to the cytokine, the reason for which is at present not understood. The cachexia-specific protein loss has also been demonstrated in human subjects in terms of nitrogen loss and increased proteolysis in skeletal muscle and liver.

The molecular mechanisms underlying cachexia have been studied using in vitro cultures of myocytes and adipocytes. For instance, the decrease in skeletal muscle protein content appears to be in part due to decreased transcription of actin and myosin genes in myocytes. Similarly, overall lipid metabolism turns catabolic, as adipocytes suppress the synthesis of lipogenic enzymes, suppress uptake of exogenous lipid and deplete their triglyceride reserves. Liver functions also are affected. For example, TNF stimulates hepatic lipogenesis, contributing to increased plasma triglyceride levels. Total liver weight is increased, which appears to be partly due to increases in total DNA and protein content. Synthesis of acute-phase reactants is induced, whereas albumin synthesis is suppressed. In addition, some of the effects leading to anorexia directly involve the central nervous system (Tracey et al., 1990).

TNF-mediated cachexia is an important complication in African trypanosomiasis, cerebral malaria, AIDS and certain cancers (Tracey and Cerami, 1991). Using animal cancer models, it has been shown that tumour-infiltrating macrophages produce TNF, which can be correlated with the development of cachexia (Moldawer et al., 1989). Also, anti-TNF antibodies have been shown to attenuate the development of cachexia in tumour models (Sherry et al., 1989). However, clinical data regarding serum TNF levels in cancer patients are limited and controversial.

AIDS Cachexia is a very common complication among AIDS patients and has been attributed to TNF found in their sera (Lahdevirta et al., 1988). HIV has been shown to stimulate monocytes to produce this protein (Merrill et al., 1989). In addition to contributing to cachexia, TNF appears to be involved in the activation of the latent phase of HIV infection, by increasing HIV expression in chronically infected T cells (Folks et al., 1989). TNF also appears to contribute to AIDS-related dementia (Price et al, 1988).

Cerebral malaria *Plasmodium falciparum* infection leads to cerebral malaria in approximately 1% of patients. In a murine model mimicking cerebral malaria, high levels of circulating TNF were found in infected mice, and use of anti-TNF antibody protected these mice from neurological complications and cachexia, without affecting parasitaemia. Together, these results suggested that this TNF contributes to the pathogenesis of cerebral malaria.

Septic shock syndrome Septic shock syndrome is caused by certain Gram-negative bacteria and manifests itself first as the Shwartzman reaction or disseminated intravascular coagulopathy, involving dehydration, metabolic acidosis, hypotension, haemorrhagic necrosis of vital organs and ultimately even death. Injection of bacterial LPS, or of TNF (which is induced by LPS), results in septic shock (Beutler and Cerami, 1988). The cytokine was found in the plasma of 36% of patients with bacterial septic shock but rarely in patients with shock resulting from other causes (Marks *et al.*, 1990). Patients with detectable TNF had a higher incidence of morbidity and mortality than did patients in whom it could not be detected.

The multiple biological effects of TNF either directly or indirectly contribute to the syndrome. Perhaps the most relevant of these effects are suppression of myocardial function and increased thrombosis, caused by increased procoagulant activity, decreased thrombomodulin, and decreased activated protein C. Other significant effects are enhanced endothelial cell adhesion and increased superoxide radical production, both of which contribute to haemorrhagic necrosis and tissue injury. In addition, capillary leak syndrome and increased eicosanoid and nitric oxide production have been demonstrated; all contribute to hypotension.

Injection of exogenous protein C has been shown to reverse some of the TNF-mediated effects. Similarly, administration of corticosteroids prior to LPS administration prevents both TNF release and LPS-mediated toxicity (Beutler *et al.*, 1986). In mice as well as in baboons, use of neutralizing anti-TNF antibodies prevented the development of septic shock induced by *Escherichia coli* (Tracey *et al.*, 1987), and by LPS (Mathison *et al.*, 1988). It also has been suggested that an anti-TNF protein (now known to be the shed form of TNF receptor), sometimes found in patient urine, may be useful in protecting against septic shock (Tracey and Cerami, 1991).

Other diseases Through its ability to modulate various immune and inflammatory functions, including the connective tissue resorption process, TNF appears to be involved in the generation of fibrotic and granulomatous lesions caused by bleomycin, silica, BCG, rheumatoid arthritis, sarcoidosis, and certain viruses (Vilcek and Palombella, 1991). It also has been suggested that, during pneumococcal meningitis, this mediator contributes to tissue damage by inducing enhanced blood–brain barrier permeability, leucocytosis in cerebrospinal fluid, and brain oedema (Saukkonen *et al.*, 1990). It has recently been demonstrated that TNF is a mediator of skin and gut lesions in graft-versus-host disease (GVHD), which is a frequent complication of allogeneic bone marrow transplantation. In experimental animal models, anti-TNF antibody could abrogate the deleterious effects of GVHD (Piguet *et al.*, 1987).

It has recently been reported that TNF modulated aberrant expression of MHC antigens. Such aberrant expression of MHC appears to be associated with autoimmune disorders. For instance, IFNγ, only when combined with TNF, induces in vitro aberrant expression of MHC II antigens by pancreatic B cells from type 1 diabetic patients (Pujol-Borrell *et al.*, 1987). Similarly, it has been observed that during various inflammatory conditions such as lupus nephritis, proximal epithelial cells in the kidney express MHC II antigens as well as TNF, suggesting that these cells participate in the pathogenesis of immune renal injury (Wuthrich *et al.*, 1990).

TNF also has been implicated in immune-mediated neurological diseases such as central demyelination (Brosnan *et al.*, 1988). TNF has been detected immunohistochemically in astrocytes and macrophages of the brains of multiple sclerosis patients (Hofman *et al.*, 1989). In experimental allergic encephalomyelitis, a murine model for multiple sclerosis, antibody inhibition of TNF and LT can prevent transfer of clinical signs of this disease (Ruddle *et al.*, 1990).

CLINICAL ROLE

In the 1890s, William Coley, a New York surgeon, used filtrates of mixed bacterial cultures (Coley's mixed toxins) to induce inflammation at the site of tumours in cancer patients and achieved complete tumour regression in 270 of 1200 patients (Coley-Nauts *et al.*, 1953). The principal active agent in Coley's mixed toxins was undoubtedly bacterial LPS, which we now know to be an inducer of TNF. Thus, this was the first documented clinical application of TNF in anticancer therapy.

The great interest in TNF as an anticancer agent, reflected by the large number of clinical trials, is based on the following abilities of this cytokine: regulation of cell growth and differentiation; toxicity towards many tumour cells; perturbation of tumour vasculature and modulation of the immune response. In addition, there is interest in using TNF for treatment of certain infectious diseases. Clinical studies should help in developing techniques for better managing its pathogenetic behaviour during syndromes such as cachexia and septic shock. Here, we will limit our discussion to the use of TNF in anticancer therapy.

rhTNF from several commercial sources has been used in single-dose and multiple-dose phase I clinical trials (Balkwill, 1989; Saks and Rosenblum, 1991). A relatively consistent pattern of side-effects, pharmacokinetics and therapeutic responses appears to be emerging. These studies have established that rhTNF can be administered in a dose range effective against cancer yet without serious side-effects such as cachexia and shock.

Pharmacokinetics Following intravenous bolus administration, rhTNF is cleared very rapidly, with a half-life of 15–30 min. Continuous intravenous infusion produces very low but steady circulating levels. The intramuscular route requires at least 150 mcg/m^2/day for TNF to be detected in the circulation, suggesting a decreased bioavailability with the change in route of administration. There is evidence that multiple administrations of the peptide do not lead to the formation of anti-TNF antibodies.

Side-effects The maximally tolerated dose of rhTNF is generally around 150-200 mcg/m^2/day. Higher doses (up to 440 mcg/m^2) are tolerated when given intravenously. The most common side-effects include fever, chills, headache and fatigue. These can be controlled with simultaneous administration of non-steroidal anti-inflammatory drugs, acetaminophen and meperidine (Saks and Rosenblum, 1991). Subcutaneous or intramuscular administration results in a severe local inflammatory reaction and thrombocytopenia. Haematological toxicity is variable.

Hypotension can become a problem at doses higher than the maximum tolerated intravenous dose. However, this can be prevented by prehydration with intravenous fluids. Neurological toxicity is infrequent. However, continuous intravenous infusion may result in seizure or transient focal neurological deficits. There is also evidence of pulmonary complications, probably because of changes in endothelial structure and permeability.

TNF therapy does not result in weight loss. Fasting serum triglyceride levels are consistently raised (Balkwill, 1989), though patients do not develop cachexia. Hypercholesterolaemia has not been seen. An acute-phase response is induced, as evidenced by the increase in serum C reactive protein, cortisol and factor VIII antigen. There is little evidence for hepatic or renal toxicity.

Responses to therapy Most phase I studies and early phase II work have not suggested a significant therapeutic effect for systemic administration of rhTNF (Figlin *et al.*, 1988; Aboulafie *et al.*, 1989; Balkwill, 1989; Saks and Rosenblum, 1991). However, these initial results should not necessarily cause pessimism, as the trials were limited in number of doses, scheduling, and sites of administration.

Administration at the tumour site has proved more promising (Taguchi, 1987; Kahn *et al.*, 1989). Such enhancement of TNF activity may be due to increase in its local concentration or to its immunomodulatory effects. Recently, rhTNF has been used intraperitoneally to treat patients suffering from malignant ascites related to gastroenteropancreatic as well as ovarian carcinomas (Raeth *et al.*, 1989; Kaufman *et al.*, 1990), with significant reduction of the ascites. In other trials, the recombinant molecule, when combined with IFNα, was successful in reducing tumours and suppressing metastases in 40% renal cell carcinoma patients. As a result, at least one commercial vendor, BASF of Germany, recently has been granted a licence to produce rhTNF for clinical use.

CONCLUSIONS

It has been said that, 'the complexity observed with TNF and other mediators is a manifestation of Nature's preoccupation with homeostasis' (Old, 1987). This is reflected in both harmful and beneficial effects of TNF, which, as described earlier, depend on several specific circumstances. These seemingly paradoxical actions have evoked comparisons of TNF to symbols of everything from ancient religion to futuristic science fiction (Old, 1990). One thing seems clear: as the molecule has been conserved throughout mammalian evolution then, despite its sometimes harmful effects, TNF must serve a useful role in the body.

Future research on TNF biology will largely reflect the desire to better control the in vivo behaviour of this cytokine. For instance, with the recent breakthroughs in TNF receptor biology, it should be possible to further study the molecular basis of TNF–TNF receptor interactions. This in turn should lead to development of compounds that may help regulate the physiological behaviour of TNF. Newer approaches in clinical studies should improve TNF's performance. For example, the adoptive transfer into cancer patients of tumour-infiltrating lymphocytes (TILs) in which the TNF gene expression is first amplified in vitro by exposure to IL-2 (Rosenberg *et al.*, 1990). An extension of this approach employs 'gene therapy', wherein the TNF gene is first inserted in TILs from a cancer patient before the cells are injected back into the patient. Early results of these trials are promising. Ultimately, the largest dividends may come from studies that employ TNF as a biological response modifier, wherein its ability to modify the behaviour of other, potentially therapeutic, cytokines is exploited.

ACKNOWLEDGEMENTS

This research was conducted in part by the Clayton Foundation for Research and New Program Development Funds from The University of Texas M. D. Anderson Cancer Center (to BBA).

REFERENCES

Aboulafie D, Miles SA, Saks SR and Mitsuyasu K (1989). Intravenous recombinant tumour necrosis factor in the treatment of AIDS-related Kaposi's sarcoma. *J AIDS*. **2**, 54–8.

Aggarwal BB (1991a). Tumour necrosis factor. In Human Cytokines: Handbook for Basic and Clinical Researchers, ed. BB Aggarwal and JU Gutterman. Cambridge, MA: Blackwell Scientific Publications 270–286.

Aggarwal BB (1991b). Structure of tumour necrosis factor and its receptor. *Biotherapy*. **3**, 113–20.

Aggarwal BB and Kohr WJ (1985a). Human tumour necrosis factor. In *Methods in enzymology* ed. G DiSabato, 441–8. New York: Academic Press.

Aggarwal BB and Vilcek J (1992). TNF: structure, function and mechanism of action. New York: Marcel Dekker Publishers,.

Aggarwal BB, Kohr WJ, Hass PE *et al.* (1985). Human tumour necrosis factor: production, purification and characterization. *J Biol Chem*. **260**, 2345–54.

Andrews JS, Berger AE and Ware CF (1990). Characterization of the receptor for tumour necrosis factor (TNF) and lymphotoxin (LT) on human T lymphocytes. TNF and LT differ in their receptor binding properties and the induction of MHC class I proteins on a human CD4+ T cell hybridoma. *J Immunol*. **114**, 2582–91.

Arakawa T and Yphantis DA (1987). Molecular weight of recombinant human tumour necrosis factor-a. *J Biol Chem*. **262**, 7484–5.

Balkwill FR (1989). Tumour necrosis factor and lymphotoxin. In *Cytokines in Cancer therapy*, ed. FR Balkwill, 54–87. New York: Oxford University Press.

Balkwill FR and Burke F (1989). The cytokine network. *Immunology Today*. **10**, 299–304.

Beutler B and Cerami A (1988). The history, properties, and biological effects of cachectin. *Biochemistry*. **27**, 7575–82.

Beutler B, Greenwald D, Hulmes JD *et al.* (1985). Identity of tumour necrosis factor and the macrophage-secreted factor cachectin. *Nature*. **316**, 552–4.

Beutler B, Krochin N, Milsark IW, Luedke C and Cerami A (1986). Control of cachectin (tumour necrosis factor) synthesis: mechanisms of endotoxin resistance. *Science*. **232**, 977–80.

Brosnan CF, Selmaj K and Raine CS (1988). Hypothesis: a role for tumour necrosis factor in immune-mediated demyelination and its relevance to multiple sclerosis. *J Neuroimmunol*. **18**, 87–94.

Broxmeyer HE, Williams DE, Lu L *et al.* (1986). The suppressive influences of human tumour necrosis factors on bone marrow hematopoietic progenitor cells from normal donors and patients with leukemia: Synergism of tumour necrosis factor and interferon-gamma. *J Immuol.* **136**, 4487–95.

Canalis E (1987). Effects of tumour necrosis factor on bone formation in vitro. *Endocrinology.* **121**, 1596–604.

Carswell EA, Old LJ, Kassel RL *et al.* (1975). An endotoxin-induced serum factor that causes necrosis of tumours. *Proc Natl Acad Sci USA.* **72**, 3666–70.

Casey ML, Cox SM, Beutler B *et al.* (1989). Cachectin/tumour necrosis factor-a formation in human desidua. Potential role of cytokines in infection-induced preterm labor. *J Clin Invest.* **83**, 430–6.

Coley-Nauts H, Fowler GA, and Bogatko FH (1953). A review of the influence of bacterial infection and bacterial products (Coley's toxins) on malignant tumour in man. *Acta Medica Scandinavica.* (**Suppl.**). **274**, 29–97.

Damonneville M, Wietzerbin V, Pancre V *et al.* (1988). Recombinant tumour necrosis factor mediates platelet cytotoxicity to *Schistosoma mansoni* larvae. *J Immunol.* **140**, 3962–5.

Davis JM, Narachi MA, Alton NK and Arakawa T (1987). Structure of human TNF-a derived from recombinant DNA. *Biochemistry.* **26**, 1322–6.

Dembic Z, Loetscher H, Gubler U *et al.* (1990). Two human TNF receptors have similar extracellular, but distinct intracellular, domain sequences. *Cytokine.* **2**, 231–7.

Dinarello CA, Cannon JG, Wolff SM *et al.* (1986). Tumour necrosis factor (cachectin) is an endogenous pyrogen and induces production of interleukin-1. *J Exp Med.* **163**, 1433–50.

Djeu JY, Blanchard DK, Halkias D and Friedman H (1986). Growth inhibition of Candida albicans by human polymorphonuclear neutrophils: activation by interferon-g and tumour necrosis factor. *J Immunol.* **137**, 2980–4.

Earl CQ, Stadel JM and Anzano MA (1990). Tumour necrosis factor-mediated biological activities involve a G-protein-dependent mechanism. *J Biol Response Mod.* **9**, 361–7.

Figlin R, Dekernion J, Sarna G, Muldower N and Saks S (1988). Phase II study of recombinant tumour necrosis factor in patients with metastatic renal cell carcinoma and malignant melanoma. *Proc Am Soc Clin Oncol.* **7**, 652.

Folks TM, Clouse KA, Justement J *et al.* (1989). Tumour necrosis factor induces expression of human deficiency virus in a chronically infected T-cell clone. *Proc Natl Acad Sci USA.* **86**, 2365–8.

Gamble JR, Harlan JM, Klebanoff SJ and Vadas MA (1985). Stimulation of the adherence of neutrophils to umbilical vein endothelium by human recombinant tumour necrosis factor. *Proc Natl Acad Sci USA.* **82**, 8667–71.

Goeddel DV, Aggarwal BB, Gray PW *et al.* (1986). Tumour necrosis factors: gene structure and biological activities. *Cold Spring Harb Symp Quant Biol.* **51**, 597–609.

Gray PW, Barrett K, Chantry D, Turner M and Fedmann M (1990). Cloning of human tumour necrosis factor (TNF) receptor cDNA and expression of recombinant soluble TNF-binding protein. *Proc Natl Acad Sci USA*. **87**, 7380–4.

Haliday EM, Ramesha CS and Ringold G (1991). TNF induces c-fos via a novel pathway requiring conversion of arachidonic acid to a lipoxygenase metabolite. *EMBO J*. **10**, 109–15.

Havell EA (1987). Production of tumour necrosis factor during murine listerosis. *J Immunol*. **139**, 4225–31.

Hofman FM, Hinton DR, Johnson K and Merrill JE (1989). Tumour necrosis factor identified in multiple sclerosis brain. *J Exp Med*. **170**, 607–12.

Ikebe T, Hirata M and Koga T (1988). Effects of human tumour necrosis factor-a and interleukin 1 on the synthesis of glycosaminoglycan and DNA in cultured rat costal chondrocytes. *J Immunol*. **140**, 827–31.

Jaatela M, Kuuselap P and Saksella E (1988). Demonstration of TNF in human amniotic fluids and supernatants of placental and decidual tissue. *Lab Invest*. **58**, 48–52.

Johnson RA, Waddelow TA, Caro J, Oliff A and Roodman GD (1989). Chronic exposure to TNF in vivo preferentially inhibits erythropoiesis in nude mice. *Blood*. **74**, 130–8.

Jones EV, Stuart DI and Walter NPC (1990). The three-dimensional structure of TNF. In *Cytokines and lipocortins in inflammation*, ed. M Melli and L Parente. Progress in Clinical and Biological Research Series, **349**, 321–327, New York: Wiley-Liss.

Kahaleh MB, Smith EA, Som Y and LeRoy EC (1988). Effect of lymphotoxin and TNF on endothelial and connective tissue cell growth and function. *Clin Immunol Immunopathol*, **49**, 261–72.

Kahn JO, Kaplan JD, Volberding PA, Ziegler JL, Saks SR AND Abrams DI (1989). Intralesional recombinant tumour necrosis factor A for AIDS-associated Kaposi's sarcoma: A randomized double-blind trial. *J AIDS*. **2**, 217–23.

Kaufman M, Schmid H, Raeth U *et al.* (1990). Therapy of ascites with tumour necrosis factor in ovarian cancer. *Geburtshilfe Frauenheilkd*. **50**, 678–82.

Kettelhut IC, Fiers W and Goldberg AL (1987). The toxic effects of tumour necrosis factor in vivo and their prevention by cyclooxygenase inhibitors. *Proc Natl Acad Sci USA*. **84**, 4273–7.

Kilbourn RG and Belloni P (1990). Endothelial cell production of nitric oxides in response to interferon G in combination with tumour necrosis factor, interleukin-1, or endotoxin. *J Natl Cancer Inst*. **82**, 772–6.

Kindler V, Sappino AP, Grau GE, Piguet PF and Vassali P (1989). The inducing role of tumour necrosis factor in the development of bactericidal granulomas during BCG infection. *Cell*. **56**, 73–140.

Klebanoff SJ, Vadas MA, Harlan JM *et al.* (1986). Stimulation of neutrophils by tumour necrosis factor. *J Immunol*. **136**, 4220–5.

Knauer MF, Longmuir KJ, Yamamoto RS, Fitzgerald TP and Granger GA (1990). Mechanism of human lymphotoxin and tumour necrosis factor induced destruction of cells in vitro: phospholipase activation and deacylation of specific-membrane phospholipids. *J Cell Physiol*. **142**, 469–79.

Kreigler M, Perez C, DeFay K *et al*. (1988). A novel form of TNF is a cell surface cytotoxic transmembrane protein. *Cell*, **52**, 45-53.

Kronke M, Schutze S, Scheurich P and Pfizenmaier K (1991). Tumour necrosis factor: signal transduction and TNF-responsive genes. In *Tumour necrosis factor: Structure, function and mechanism of action*, ed. BB Aggarwal and J Vilcek, 189-216 New York: Marcel Dekker Publishers.

Lahdevirta J, Maury CP, Teppo AM and Repo H (1988). Elevated levels of circulating cachectin/tumour necrosis factor in patients with acquired immunodeficiency syndrome. *Am J Med*. **85**, 289–91.

Marino MW, Feld LJ, Jaffe EA *et al*. (1991). Phosphorylation of the proto-oncogene product eukaryotic initiation factor 4E is a common cellular response to tumour necrosis factor. *J Biol Chem*. **266**, 2685-8.

Marks JD. Berman-Marks C, Luce JM *et al*. (1990). Plasma tumour necrosis factor in patients with septic shock: mortality rate, incidence of ARDS, and effects of methylprednisolone administration. *Am Rev Respir Dis*. **141**, 94–7.

Marquet RL, De Bruin RWF, Fiers W and Jeekel J (1987). Antitumour activity of mouse TNF on colon cancer in rats is promoted by recombinant rat interferon. *Int J Cancer* **40**, 550–3.

Mathison JC, Wolfson E and Ulevitch RJ (1988). Participation of tumour necrosis factor in the mediation of gram negative bacterial lipopolysaccharide-induced injury in rabbits. *J Clin Invest*. **81**, 2925–37.

Matsushima K, Morishita K, Yoshimura T *et al*. (1988). Molecular cloning of a human monocyte-derived neutrophil chemotactic factor (MDNCF) and the induction of MDNCF mRNA by interleukin-1 and tumour necrosis factor. *J Exp Med*. **167**, 1883–93.

McCann SM, Rettori V, Milenkovic L, Jurcovicova J and Gonzalez MC (1990). Role of monokines in control of anterior pituitery hormone release. In *Circulating regulatory factors and neuroendocrine function*, ed. JC Porter and D Jezova, 315–329. New York: Plenum Press.

Merrill JE, Koyanagi Y and Chen IS (1989). Interleukin-1 and tumour necrosis factor-a can be induced from mononuclear phagocytes by human immunodeficiency virus type 1 binding to the CD4 receptor. *J Virol*. **63**, 4404–8.

Ming WJ, Bersani L and Mantovani A (1987). Tumour necrosis factor is chemotactic for monocytes and polymorphonuclear leukocytes. *J Immunol*. **138**, 1469–74.

Moldawer LL, Sherry B, Lowry SF and Cerami A (1989). Endogenous cachectin/tumour necrosis factor-a production contributes to experimental cancer-associated cachexia. *Cancer Surveys*. **8**, 853–9.

Mosselmans R, Hepburn A, Dumont JE, Fiers W and Galand P (1988). Endocytic pathway of recombinant murine tumour necrosis factor in L-929 cells. *J Immunol.* **141**, 3096–100.

Mundy GR, Roodman GD, Bonewald LF, Yoneda T and Sabatini M (1991). Effects of tumour necrosis factor (TNF) and lymphotoxin (LT) on bone cells and calcium metabolism. In *Tumour necrosis factor: structure, function and mechanism of action.* ed. J Vilcek and BB Aggarwal, 483–98. New York: Marcel Dekker Publishing Co.

Mushtaha AA, Schmalsteig FC, Hughes TK Jr. *et al.* (1989). Chemokinetic agents for monocytes in human milk: possible role of tumour necrosis factor-a. *Pediatr Res.* **25**, 629–33.

Nathan CF (1987). Neutrophil activation on biological surfaces. Massive secretion of hydrogen peroxide in response to products of macrophages and lymphocytes. *J Clin Invest.* **80**, 1550–60.

Neale ML, Fiera RA and Matthews N (1988). Involvement of phospholipase A2 in tumour cell killing by tumour necrosis factor. *Immunology.* **64**, 81–5.

Neta R (1990). Radioprotection and therapy of radiation injury with cytokines. *Prog Clin Biol Res.* **352**, 471–8.

O'Malley WE, Achinstein B and Shear MJ (1962). Action of bacterial polysaccharide on tumours. II. Damage of sarcoma 37 by serum of mice treated with Serratia marcescens polysaccharide, and induced tolerance. *J Natl Cancer Inst.* **29**, 1169–75.

Old. LJ (1987). Introduction. In *Tumour necrosis factor and related cytotoxins,* CIBA Foundation Symposium, No. 131, pp. 1-2, Chichester,: Wiley and Sons.

Old LJ (1990). Tumour necrosis factor. In *Tumour necrosis factor, structure, mechanism of action, role in disease and therapy*, ed. B Bonavida,and G Granger, 1–30. Basel: Karger Publishing Co.

Palombella VJ and Vilcek J (1989). Mitogenic and cytotoxic actions of tumour necrosis factor in BALB/c 3T3 cells. *J Biol Chem.* **264**, 18128–36.

Pennica D, Nedwin GE, Hayflick JF *et al.* (1984). Human TNF: Precursor structure, expression and homology to lymphotoxin. *Nature.* **312**, 724–9.

Perez C, Albert I, DeFay K, Zachariades N, Gooding L and Kriegler M (1990). A nonsecretable cell surface mutant of TNF kills by cell-to-cell contact. *Cell.* **63**, 251–8.

Perlmutter DH. Dinarello CA, Punsal PI and Colten HR (1986). Cachectin/tumour necrosis factor regulates hepatic acute-phase gene expression. *J. Clin. Invest.* **78**, 1349–54 .

Piguet PF, Grau GE, Allet B and Vassalli P (1987). Tumour necrosis factor/cachectin is an effector of skin and gut lesions of the acute phase of graft-versus-host disease. *J Exp Med.* **166**, 1280–9.

Porteu F and Nathan C (1990). Shedding of tumour necrosis factor receptors by activated human neutrophils. *J Exp Med.* **172**, 599–607.

Price RW, Brew B, Sidtis J *et al.* (1988). The brain in AIDS: Central nervous system HIV-1 infection and AIDS dementia complex. *Science.* **239**, 586–92.

Pujol-Borrell R, Todd I, Doshi M *et al.* (1987). HLA class II induction in human islet cells by interferon-g plus tumour necrosis factor or lymphotoxin. *Nature.* **326**, 304–5.

Radeke HH, Meier B, Topley N *et al.* (1990). Interleukin 1-a and tumour necrosis factor-a induce oxygen radical production in mesangial cells. *Kidney International.* **37**, 767–75

Raeth U. Schmid H, Hofman J *et al.* (1989). Intraperitoneal (i.p.) application of recombinant human tumour necrosis factor (rHuTNF) as an effective palliative treatment of malignant ascites from ovarian and gastroenteropancreatic carcinomas. *Proc Am Soc Clin Oncol.* **8**, 181.

Remick DG, Strieter RM, Eskandari MK *et al.* (1990). Role of tumour necrosis factor-a in lipopolysaccharide-induced pathologic alterations. *Am J Pathol.* **136**, 49–60.

Roodman GD, Bird A, Hultzer D and Montgomery W (1987). Tumour necrosis factor-a and hematopoietic progenitors: Effects of tumour necrosis factor on the growth of erythroid progenitors CFU-E and BFU-E and the hematopoietic cell lines K562, HL60, and HEL cells. *Exp Hematol.* **15**, 928–35.

Rosenberg SA, Aebersold P, Cornetta K *et al.* (1990). Gene transfer into humans– immunotherapy of patients with advanced melanoma, using tumour-infiltrating lymphocytes modified by retroviral gene transduction. *N Engl J Med.* **323**, 570–8.

Ruddle NH, Bergman CM, Lingenheld EG *et al.* (1990). An antibody to lymphotoxin and tumour necrosis factor prevents transfer of experimental allergic encephalomyelitis. *J Exp Med.* **172**, 1193–200.

Saks S and Rosenblum MG (1991). Recombinant human TNF-a: Preclinical studies and results from early clinical trials. In *Tumour necrosis factor: structure, function and mechanism of action.* ed. J Vilcek and BB Aggarwal, 567–87. New York: Marcel Dekker Publishing Co.

Salmon SE, Soehnlen B and Scuderi P (1985). Natural product-resistant leukemia and myeloma cells exhibit sensitivity to recombinant tumour necrosis factor. *Blood.* **66 (suppl. 1)**, 29.

Saukkonen K. Sande S, Cioffe C *et al.* (1990). The role of cytokines in the generation of inflammation and tissue damage in experimental gram-positive meningitis. *J Exp Med.* **171**, 439–48.

Scholz W and Altman A (1989). Synergistic induction of interleukin 2 receptor (TAC) expression on YT cells by interleukin 1 or tumour necrosis factor A in combination with cAMP inducing agent. *Cell Signal.* **1**, 367–75.

Schutze S, Nottrott S, Pfizenmaier K and Kronke M (1990). Tumour necrosis factor signal transduction. Cell-type-specific activation and translocation of protein kinase C. *J Immunol.* **144**, 2604–8.

Selman K and Raine CS (1988). Tumour necrosis factor mediates myelin and oligodendrocyte damage in vitro. *Am Neurol.* **23**, 339–46.

Shalaby MR, Aggarwal BB, Rinderknecht E *et al.* (1985). Activation of human polymorphonuclear neutrophil functions by interferon-gamma and tumour necrosis factors. *J Immunol.* **135**, 2069–73.

Shemer-Avni Y, Wallach D and Sarov I (1988). Inhibition of Chlamydia trachomatis growth by recombinant tumour necrosis factor. *Infection and Immunity.* **56**, 2503–6.

Sherry BA, Gelin J. Fong Y *et al.* (1989). Anticachectin/tumour necrosis factor-a antibodies attenuate development of cachexia in tumour models. *FASEB J.* **3**, 1956–62.

Slungaard A, Vercellotti GM, Walker G *et al.* (1990). Tumour necrosis factor/cachectin stimulates eosinophil oxidant production and toxicity towards human endothelium. *J Exp Med.* **171**, 2025–41.

Smith MR, Munger WE, Kung H-F, Takacs L and Durum S.K (1990). Direct evidence for an intracellular role for tumour necrosis factor-a: Microinjection of TNF kills target cells. *J Immunol.* **144**, 162–9.

Spies T, Blanck G. Bresnahan M, Sands J and Strominger JL.(1989). A new cluster of genes within the human major histocompatibility complex. *Science.* **243**, 214–17.

Sprang SR (1990). The divergent receptors for TNF. *Trends Biochem Sci.* **15**, 366–8.

Spriggs D, Deutsch S and Kufe DW (1991). Genomic structure, induction, and production of tumour necrosis factor-a. In *TNF: structure, function and mechanism of action*, ed. J Vilcek and BB Aggarwal, 3-34. New York, NY: Marcel Dekker Publishing Co.

Spriggs DW, Sherman ML, Imamura K *et al.* (1990). Phosphilipase A2 activation and autoinduction of tumour necrosis factor gene expression by tumour necrosis factor. *Cancer Res.* **50**, 7101–7.

Sugarman BJ, Aggarwal BB, Hass PE *et al.* (1985). Recombinant TNF: Effects on proliferation of normal and transformed cells in vitro. *Science*, **230**, 943–5.

Taguchi T (1987). Recombinant human tumour necrosis factor (rhu-TNF) phase–I and early phase–II study. *Proc Am Soc Clin Oncol.* **6**, 233.

Taverne J, Tavernier J, Fiers W *et al.* (1987). Recombinant tumour necrosis factor inhibits malaria parasites in vivo but not in vitro. *Clin Exp Immunol.* **67**, 1–4.

Titus RG, Sherry B and Cerami A (1989). Tumour necrosis factor plays a protective role in experimental murine cutaneous leishmaniasis. *J Exp Med.* **170**, 2097–104.

Tovey MG (1988). The expression of cytokines in the organs of normal individuals: Role in homeostasis; a review. *J Biol Regul Homeost Agents.* **2**, 87–92.

Tracey KJ and Cerami A (1991). Pleiotropic effects of TNF in infection and neoplasia: Beneficial, inflammatory, catabolic, or injurious. In *TNF: structure, function and mechanism of action.* ed. J Vilcek and BB Aggarwal, 431–52. New York: Marcel Dekker Publishing Co.

Tracey KJ, Lowry SF, Beutler B *et al.* (1986). Cachectin/tumour necrosis factor mediates changes of skeletal muscle plasma membrane potential. *J Exp Med.* **164**, 1368–73.

Tracey KJ, Fong Y, Hesse DG *et al.* (1987). Anti-cachectin/TNF monoclonal antibodies prevent septic shock during lethal bacteremia. *Nature.* **330**, 662–4.

Tracey KJ, Morgello S, Koplin B *et al.* (1990). Metabolic effects of cachectin/tumour necrosis factor are modified by site of production. Cachectin/tumour necrosis factor-secreting tumour in skeletal muscle induces chronic cachexia, while implantation in brain induces predominantly acute anorexia. *J Clin Invest.* **86**, 2014–24.

Vilcek J and Palombella VJ (1991). TNFs as growth factors. In *Tissue necrosis factor: structure, function and mechanism of action.* ed. J.Vilcek and BB Aggarwal, 269–88. New York: Marcel Dekker Publishing Co.

Wirth JJ and Kirszenbaum F (1988). Recombinant tumour necrosis factor enhances macrophage destruction of Trypanosoma cruzi in the presence of bacterial endotoxin. *J Immunol.* **141**, 286–8.

Wong GHW and Goeddel DV (1986). Tumour necrosis factors A and B inhibit virus replication and synergize with interferons. *Nature.* **323**, 819–22.

Wong GHW, Krowka JF. Stites DP and Goeddel DV (1988). In vitro anti-HIV activities of TNF-a and interferon-g. *J Immunol.* **140**, 120–4.

Wong GHW, Elwell JH, Oberley LW and Goeddel DV (1989). Manganous superoxide dismutase is essential for cellular resistance to cytotoxicity of tumour necrosis factor. *Cell.* **58**, 923–31.

Wuthrich RP, Glimcher LH, Yui MA *et al.* (1990). MHC class II antigen presentation and tumour necrosis factor in renal tubular epithelial cells. *Kidney International.* **37**, 783–92.

Yoshimura T, Sone S and Ogura T (1990). Membrane perturbation as a possible cytotoxic mechanism of TNF and interferons. In *Tumour necrosis factor: structure, mechanism of action, role in disease and therapy.* ed. B Bonavida and G Granger, 70–6. Basel: Karger Publishing Co.

Zhang YH, Lin JX, Yip YK and Vilcek (1988). Enhancement of cAMP levels and of protein kinase activity by tumour necrosis factor and interleukin-1 in human fibroblasts: Role in the induction of interleukin 6. *Proc Natl Acad Sci USA.* **85**, 6802–5.

11

THE CYTOKINE NETWORK

M. K. BRENNER

INTRODUCTION

Previous chapters in this book have described how individual cytokines affect cells, cell lines, or whole organisms. These 'pharmacological effects' may have rather little to do with the physiological importance of cytokines in a normally functioning organism. It is rare that a single cytokine will be released following any physiological stimuli in vivo. Instead, the influence of cytokines in the animal as a whole relates to their ability to behave as a highly interactive network, in which entry of any one cytokine into the system is associated with changes in the production of and the response to many other cytokines. One of the purposes of this chapter is to describe some of the characteristics of this cytokine network.

We will also show how information exchange within the network has some of the characteristics of a language. The cytokine proteins represent the vocabulary, the order in which the cytokines are produced forms the syntax, while the influence of context on the outcome of target cell exposure means the cytokine network even has its own semantics and semiotics.

Finally, we will illustrate how the physiological importance of the network has major implications for the therapeutic use of cytokines. Because the specificity and efficacy of cytokine action depends on mobilization of particular components of a complex and interactive network, administration of a single cytokine will rarely, if ever, produce as great or as well directed a therapeutic benefit as a combination of the agents administered in the correct sequence and with the correct timing.

Unfortunately, the dictates of clinical trial design mean that most studies to date have only been able to investigate the activity of single agents. We should not, therefore, be disappointed by the limited therapeutic benefits so far reported with individual cytokines, such as IL-2, IFNα and GM-CSF. Instead we should be pleasantly surprised that such comparatively feeble and constrained attempts to imitate or modify so complex and interactive a network ever produce any benefit at all. As this chapter will try to illustrate, the imminent introduction of cytokine combinations into clinical trials should mean that the therapeutic effects of cytokines will ultimately be shown to greatly exceed their modest beginnings as individual agents.

THE STRUCTURE AND COMPLEXITY OF THE CYTOKINE NETWORK

The original concept of cytokine action was that each protein acted on one or more cell types in a given stage of differentiation, to induce or inhibit proliferation and/or further differentiation. Many examples of such cytokine actions have been described in the preceding chapters of this book. However, with the possible exception of those cytokines that act strictly as lineage restricted growth factors (e.g. erythropoietin and G-CSF), the action of a cytokine on a given cell almost invariably induces the release of a range of secondary cytokines. These may have additive, synergistic or even competitive actions with the first cytokine and may act on entirely different target cells (see below). Moreover, if a cytokine (such as IL-1) acts on a range of different target cells, the pattern of secondary cytokine induction may be separate in each.

This complex network effect particularly dominates the actions of cytokines such as IL-1, IL-2, IL-6 and TNF, which are involved in the inflammatory and immune responses.

Interleukin-2 as an example of a network cytokine

Interleukin-2 acts primarily on receptor-bearing lymphocytes to induce cellular proliferation and enhance activation. These activation events include the synthesis and release of a large number of secondary cytokines, which in turn modify the growth of secondary target cells. For example, the cytokines induced by IL-2 include GM-CSF and IL-3, which are growth factors active on the haemopoietic system. As one would predict, therefore, IL-2 infusion may be followed by an increase in circulating neutrophil numbers. Such an event is seen if IL-2 is administered after myelosuppressive chemotherapy or following marrow transplantation. It is important to emphasize that this myelostimulation takes place even though IL-2 itself has no direct effect on haemopoietic progenitor cell growth. Instead, the effects on neutrophils are entirely dependent on the operation of a network effect and would not be predictable from the original target cell range or from patterns of IL-2 receptor expression. But because of the extent of the cytokine network, the consequences of IL-2 infusion for the haematopoietic system may be more complex. The action of IL-2 on its primary lymphocyte target also induces release of TNF and IFNγ. These two cytokines have precisely the opposite effects on marrow progenitor cells to IL-3 and GM-CSF and may suppress myeloid growth and differentiation. During some IL-2 dose regimens these inhibitory effects dominate and IL-2 actually produces a fall in neutrophil and platelet counts.

The network has one further layer of complexity. Many of the secondary cytokines induced by IL-2 themselves induce tertiary cytokines, which again may have actions conflicting with the activities of the primary or secondary agents. To extend the example quoted above, TNF as a secondary cytokine directly inhibits the growth of marrow progenitor cells, but induces 'tertiary' cytokines from marrow stromal cells. These include G-CSF, a stimulator of myeloid cell proliferation and differentiation.

It can readily be seen that one consequence of the multilayered complexity of the cytokine network means that the outcome of administering even a single cytokine may depend on the cytokine dose, duration of administration and on the state of the primary and secondary target organs (see below).

Limiting the cytokine network

Because many cytokines induce a range of secondary cytokines, and because many of these agents in turn induce tertiary cytokines, the obvious puzzle is why any trigger to the system does not cause it to behave as an uncontrolled amplification cascade and produce lethal consequences. In part, these undesirable cascade effects are prevented by in-built damping mechanisms. Thus, the network elicited in response to any cytokine contains homeostatic as well as activating cytokines. Administration of IL-2, for example, also induces IL-4, a cytokine that down-regulates production of other cytokine proteins and helps to shut down the network once the triggering stimuli have passed (see below). A number of other such inhibitory cytokines have been identified, including transforming growth factor alpha (TGFα) and β interferon, and these may work by enhancing degradation of cytokine mRNA or by dephosphorylating activated messenger proteins or by phosphorylating inhibitory cellular molecules. The inhibitory component of the network works in conjunction with other down-regulation mechanisms, which include production of cytokine binding proteins (see Chapter 10), soluble forms of cytokine receptor or anticytokine antibodies.

Implications of the cytokine network

The potency and the extent of the cytokine network have three implications for the optimal design of therapeutic regimens incorporating cytokines. First, the consequences of administering even a single cytokine may be far more wide ranging than anticipated and some of these network effects may actually be responsible for many of the apparently beneficial and for many of the adverse effects of the initial cytokine used. For example, the TNF induced by IL-2 may be of benefit by contributing to the antitumour activity of IL-2, but it may also be harmful in the short term, as it probably contributes to the capillary leak syndrome and hypotension associated with prolonged infusion of IL-2. Secondly, it may be possible to increase the therapeutic index of cytokine infusion by blocking unwanted components of the network – for example, using anti-TNF antibodies to reduce the hypotension and capillary leak associated with IL-2 infusion. Finally, it may be possible to prolong or abbreviate the effect of a cytokine by respectively blocking or infusing homeostatic cytokines such as IL-4 or TGFβ.

It is likely, therefore, that future cytokine regimens will include not only the therapeutic cytokines under study, but also homeostatic cytokines and/or cytokine antibodies, which will more tightly focus the cytokine network, so that the desired effects are produced predominantly only on the targeted cells or organ.

THE LANGUAGE OF CYTOKINES

An understanding of the way in which cytokines and the networks in which they operate can produce so varied a range of effects can be gleaned by considering the proteins as part of a language. Individual cytokine proteins (the 'vocabulary') convey little information per se, while random ordering of the vocabulary produces a confused or meaningless message (Fig. 11.1(a)). The proteins instead have to be organized into a formal structure, in terms of sequence and intensity, by the imposition of a syntax (Fig. 11.1(b)). But the information conveyed and the response elicited by even a syntactically correct cytokine 'sentence' is context dependent (Fig. 11.1(c)) and will be affected by the state of differentiation and activation of the target cells and by the overall environment in which the cytokine message is received.

(a) VOCABULARY = CYTOKINE PROTEINS

IS CRAB MAN THE EATING

(b) SYNTAX = CYTOKINE SEQUENCE

THE MAN IS EATING THE CRAB

(c) CONTEXT = EVENTS PRECEDING EXPOSURE

THE CRAB IS CONTAMINATED.

THE MAN IS EATING THE CRAB

Fig. 11.1. The language of the cytokine network.

Examples of the importance of cytokine syntax

A large number of cytokines modify the growth and differentiation of haemopoietic progenitor cells. Some act on early progenitors (e.g. Steele factor, IL-1, TNF and IL-6) while others act on more committed progenitors (e.g. IL-3, GM-CSF) or on fully committed lineage restricted cells (e.g. G-CSF, M-CSF, IL-5).

The importance of cytokine syntax can be seen if the effects of cytokines from these different groups are examined individually or when they are combined in different order. These effects are readily demonstrated during periods of profound marrow regeneration. Following bone marrow transplantation, for example, the engrafting marrow initially regenerates predominantly by expansion of the early progenitor compartment. Expansion is followed by progressive differentiation to committed precursors, which then mature into the formed elements of the blood. Exogenous cytokines will individually facilitate proliferation and differentiation of cells at given stages of development, but no single cytokine can convey the multiplicity of information required by all the components in a regenerating marrow. Thus, administration of late acting cytokines such as G-CSF following BMT makes a minimal impact on the rate with which neutrophils re-appear. There are simply too few progenitors in an appropriate late stage of differentiation to produce a major clinical response. Cytokines that act earlier in marrow

(a)

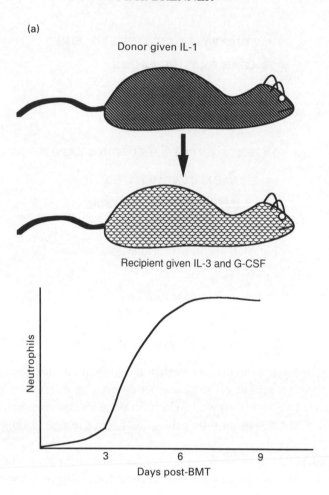

Donor given IL-1

Recipient given IL-3 and G-CSF

Fig. 11.2(a). The importance of cytokine syntax.

development, such as IL-3, are similarly ineffective – though for a different reason. These cytokines may expand early progenitors but do not instruct them to progress through further differentiation into mature formed elements.

Only when early- and late-acting cytokines are combined is their ability to augment marrow proliferation and maturation evident. If marrow is obtained from mice pretreated with IL-1, and then transplanted into mice, which are then given IL-3, followed by G-CSF, the results are dramatic (Fig. 11.2a). In the presence of these later-acting factors, the 'early factor'-treated marrow will repopulate the recipient mouse in just 3 or 4 days. The importance of cytokine syntax is readily shown in this model by changing the order of the cytokines administered. If the donor mouse is pretreated with a late-acting

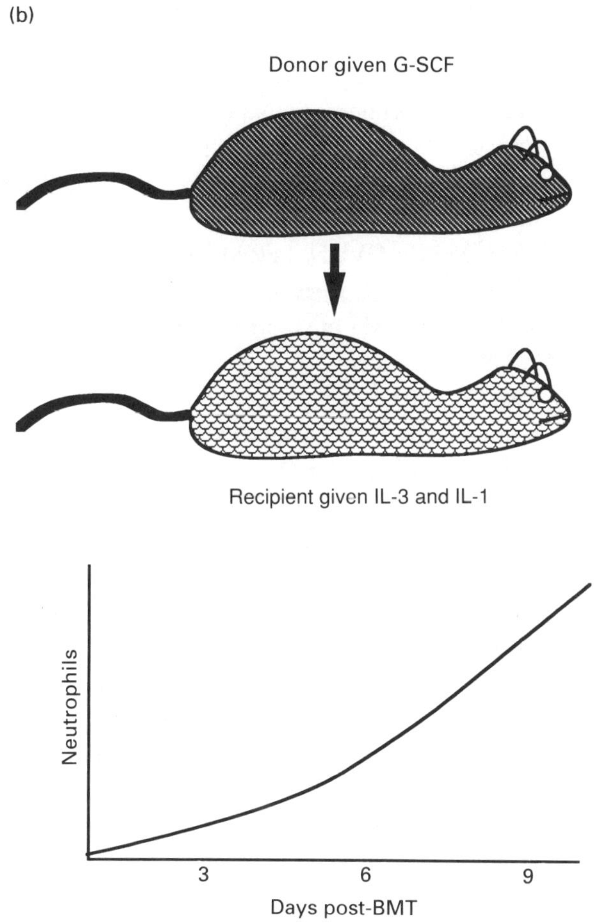

(b)

Donor given G-SCF

Recipient given IL-3 and IL-1

Fig. 11.2(b). The importance of cytokine syntax.

factor and the recipient mouse is given early-acting agents, then the extremely rapid marrow recovery is not seen, and regeneration is only slightly faster than in control animals (Fig. 11.2(b)).

Examples of the importance of cytokine context

Interleukin-2: enhancer or inhibitor of T cell function? The importance of considering context in assessing the likely impact of a cytokine can be illustrated by the effects of IL-2 on the immune system. IL-2 is best known for its ability to activate T cells and natural killer (NK) cells and to induce

183

these cells to release cytokines. In some contexts, however, IL-2 may not stimulate the immune system but may actually inhibit it.

Graft-versus-host disease (GVHD) following bone marrow transplantation is produced when alloreactive donor T lymphocytes recognize host antigens and become activated. They release cytokines, including TNF, which in turn recruit other cytotoxic effector cells from the immune system. Administration of a lymphocyte growth factor, such as IL-2 after allogeneic BMT would therefore be fuelling an already inflammatory mixture and would be predicted to accelerate and exacerbate GVHD. Indeed, precisely such an effect can be produced in mice given IL-2 after receiving an allogeneic BMT. However, the overall effects of IL-2 after BMT are more subtle, as IL-2, paradoxically, also induces specific unresponsiveness to host alloantigens. This effect can be shown in two ways. If patients receiving autologous BMT are treated with cyclosporin-A, a drug that prevents lymphocyte release of and response to IL-2, then it is possible to induce GVHD, even though no alloreactive T cells were present in the original marrow. In other words, while IL-2 may augment the growth and proliferation of alloreactive T cells, it can also prevent the de novo appearance of these cells by helping the development of T cell tolerance to self antigens in the thymus during the period of lymphoid regeneration which follows BMT. Similarly, there is now evidence that IL-2 can even induce anergy in the mature alloreactive T cells which are transferred after allogeneic BMT and which would otherwise produce severe GVHD. If mice receive a marrow allograft together with syngeneic T-lymphocyte-depleted marrow, administration of IL-2 now renders donor T cells specifically unresponsive to recipient alloantigens. This effect, of course, is precisely the opposite to that conventionally expected from giving IL-2 after allogeneic BMT.

Thus, exposure to host histocompatibility antigens and IL-2 in one context may potentiate GVHD, while in a second, closely related context, the same cytokine may inhibit T cell responsiveness to alloantigens and actually abrogate GVHD.

Interleukin-4: enhancer or inhibitor of cytotoxic effector function?
Interleukin-4 is a cytokine with pleiotropic effects on the immune system. Clinically, most interest revolves around its ability to enhance the cytotoxicity of CD3+ CD8+ activated killer (AK) cells. The hope has been that IL-4 would augment the therapeutic effects of IL-2-induced AK cells in the eradication of malignant disease. This faith may be misplaced. While it is true that concomitant administration of IL-2 and IL-4 can enhance T-cytotoxic cell activity, the effects of sequential exposure to the cytokine may be quite different. IL-4 is one of the secondary cytokines induced when lymphocytes are exposed to IL-2. Under these conditions, IL-4 behaves not as an enhancer

of IL-2 driven cytotoxic activity but as a homeostatic regulator. IL-4 can de-phosphorylate the second messenger proteins, which are phosphorylated in response to cell activation by IL-2. As a consequence, IL-4 shortens the half-life of IL-2-induced AK cells and diminishes their release of stimulatory cytokines such as TNF and IFNγ. In other words, IL-4 makes a major contribution to limiting the positive feedback potential of IL-2 (see above).

Thus, whether IL-4 enhances or inhibits IL-2-dependent cytotoxicity is context dependent and is affected not only by the state of target cell activation but also by the relative timing of exposure to each cytokine.

Tumour necrosis factor: tumour inhibitor or tumour growth factor? TNF was so named because of its capacity to kill or inhibit the growth of a variety of tumour cells in animal and human in vitro model systems. While this capability undoubtedly exists, it is also true that TNF can act as a tumour growth factor. This effect appears particularly important in certain malignancies derived from cells for which TNF is normally a growth stimulatory cytokine. For example, TNF is a growth/differentiation factor for normal B lymphocytes. It is also an (autocrine) growth factor for at least two B-cell-derived malignancies, hairy-cell leukaemia and chronic B lymphocytic leukaemia. The survival of cells from these malignancies is prolonged by tumour necrosis factor and, indeed, in some cases the tumour cells may actually proliferate following exposure to this nominally inhibitory cytokine.

These effects illustrate how important it is to consider context in evaluating the likely outcome of a cytokine's activity in any specific instance, and that it is essential to avoid being beguiled simply by a name.

CONCLUSION

An understanding of the physiology of cytokines and the ability to make use of their full therapeutic potential will come only when we have learned more about the ways in which these agents interact and when we can better comprehend the information conveyed by complex mixtures of cytokine proteins. Once this understanding has been achieved, there is now good reason to believe that it will be followed rapidly by major advances in our ability to prevent and treat a multiplicity of currently intractable disorders.

FURTHER READING

Balkwill FR and Burke F (1989). The cytokine network. *Immunology Today.* **10**, 299-304.

Lang RA and Burgess AW (1990). Autocrine growth factors and tumourigenic transformation. *Immunology Today*. **11**, 244-9.

Metcalf D (1989). The molecular control of cell division, differentiation commitment and maturation in heamopoietic stem cells. *Nature*. **339**, 27-30.

Metcalf D. (1991). Control of granulocytes and monocytes; molecular, cellular and clinical aspects. *Science*. **254**, 529–33.

Paul WE (1989). Pleiotropy and redundancy: T cell-derived lymphokines in the immune response. *Cell*. **57**, 521-4.

Paul WE (1991). Interleukin-4: A prototypic immunoregulatory lymphokine. *Blood*. **77**, 1859-70.

Sporn MB and Roberts AB (1989). Peptide growth factors are multifunctional. *Nature*. **332**, 217-19.

INDEX

INDEX